前　言

《循证针灸临床实践指南》包括：带状疱疹、贝尔面瘫、抑郁症、中风后假性球麻痹、偏头痛、颈椎病、慢性便秘、腰痛、原发性痛经、坐骨神经痛、失眠、成人支气管哮喘、肩周炎、膝关节炎、急慢性胃炎、过敏性鼻炎、突发性耳聋、三叉神经痛、糖尿病周围神经病变、单纯性肥胖病等病症的循证针灸临床实践指南。

本部分为《循证针灸临床实践指南》的失眠部分。

本部分受国家中医药管理局指导与委托。

本部分由中国针灸学会提出。

本部分由中国针灸学会标准化工作委员会归口。

本部分起草单位：中国中医科学院针灸研究所。

本部分主要起草人：杨金洪、胡静、王兵、张宁、姜爱平、曹建萍、尹红红、杨逢春。

本部分专家组成员：刘保延、赵宏、武晓冬、房繁恭、赵吉平、刘志顺、吴泰相、吴中朝、刘炜宏、梁繁荣、张维、杨金生、文碧玲、余曙光、郭义、杨骏、赵京生、杨华元、储浩然、石现、王富春、王麟鹏、贾春生、余晓阳、高希言、常小荣、张洪涛、吕明庄、王玲玲、宣丽华、翟伟、岗卫娟、王昕、董国锋、王芳。

引　言

　　《循证针灸临床实践指南》是根据针灸临床优势，针对特定临床情况，参照古代文献、名医经验以及现代最佳临床研究证据，结合患者价值观和意愿，系统研制的帮助临床医生和患者做出恰当针灸处理的指导性意见。

　　《循证针灸临床实践指南》制定的总体思路是：在针灸实践与临床研究的基础上，遵循循证医学的理念与方法，紧紧围绕针灸临床的特色优势，综合专家经验、目前最佳证据以及患者价值观，将国际公认的证据质量评价与推荐方案分级的规范与古代、前人、名老针灸专家临床证据相结合，并将临床研究证据与大范围专家共识相结合，旨在制定出能保障针灸临床疗效和安全性、并具有科学性与实用性的可有效指导针灸临床实践的指导性意见。

　　在《循证针灸临床实践指南》的制定过程中，各专家组共同参与，还完成了国家标准《针灸临床实践指南制定与评估规范》（以下简称《规范》）的送审稿。《规范》参照了国际上临床实践指南制定的要求和经验，根据中国国情以及针灸的发展状况，对《循证针灸临床实践指南》制定的组织、人员、过程、采用证据质量评价、推荐方案等级划分、专家共识形成方式、制定与更新的内容和时间等都进行了规范。这些规范性要求在《循证针灸临床实践指南》制定中都得到了充分考量与完善。《规范》与《循证针灸临床实践指南》相辅相成，《规范》是《循证针灸临床实践指南》制定的指导，《循证针灸临床实践指南》又是《规范》适用性的验证实例。

　　《循证针灸临床实践指南》推荐等级主要采用世界卫生组织（WHO）等推荐的GRADE（Grading of Recommendations Assessment，Development and Evaluation）系统，即推荐分级的评价、制定与评估的系统，其中推荐等级分为强推荐与弱推荐两级。强推荐的方案是估计变化可能性较小、个性化程度低的方案，而弱推荐方案则是估计变化可能性较大、个性化程度高、患者价值观差异大的方案。对于古代文献和名医经验的证据质量评价，目前课题组还在进一步研制中，《循证针灸临床实践指南》仅将古代文献和名医经验作为证据之一附列在现代证据后面，供《循证针灸临床实践指南》使用者参考。

　　2008年，在WHO西太区的项目资助下，由中国中医科学院牵头、中国针灸学会标准化工作委员会组织完成了针灸治疗带状疱疹、贝尔面瘫、抑郁症、中风后假性球麻痹和偏头痛5种病症的指南研制工作。在这5种病症的指南研制过程中，课题组初步提出了《循证针灸临床实践指南》的研究方法和建议，建立了《循证针灸临床实践指南》的体例、研究模式与技术路线。2010年12月，《临床病症中医临床实践指南·针灸分册》由中国中医药出版社正式出版发行。

　　2009年至2013年，在国家中医药管理局立项支持下，中国针灸学会标准化工作委员会又先后分3批启动了15种病症的指南研制工作。为了保证《循证针灸临床实践指南》高质量地完成，在总课题组的组织下，由四川大学华西医院吴泰相教授在京举办2次GRADE方法学培训会议，全国11家临床及科研单位的100多位学员接受了培训。随后，总课题组又组织了15个疾病临床指南制定课题组和1个方法学课题组中的17位研究人员，赴华西医院循证医学中心接受了为期3个月的Meta分析和GRADE方法学专题培训，受训研究人员系统学习并掌握了GRADE系统证据质量评价和推荐意见形成的方法。

　　本次出版的《循证针灸临床实践指南》共有20个部分，包括对2010年版5部分指南的修订再版和 2013 年完成的 15 部分指南的首次出版。《循证针灸临床实践指南》的适用对象为从事针灸临床与科研的专业人员。

《循证针灸临床实践指南》的证据质量分级和推荐强度等级如下：

◇证据质量分级

证据质量高：A

证据质量中：B

证据质量低：C

证据质量极低：D

◇推荐强度等级

支持使用某项干预措施的强推荐：1

支持使用某项干预措施的弱推荐：2

《循证针灸临床实践指南》的编写，凝聚着全国针灸标准化科研人员和管理人员的辛勤汗水，是参与研制各方集体智慧的结晶，是辨证论治的个体化诊疗模式与循证医学有机结合的创造性探索。《循证针灸临床实践指南》在研制过程中，得到了兰州大学循证医学中心杨克虎教授、陈耀龙博士以及北京大学循证医学中心詹思延教授在方法学上的大力支持和帮助，在此深表感谢。同时，还要感谢国家中医药管理局政策法规与监督司领导的热心指导与大力支持；此外，还要感谢各位专家的通力合作；在《循证针灸临床实践指南》的出版过程中，中国中医药出版社表现出了很高的专业水平，在此一并致谢。

摘　　要

1　治疗原则

针灸治疗失眠应在脏腑辨证的基础上，按患者主诉症状进行针对性治疗。以整体睡眠质量、睡眠时间、日间觉醒状态为主要障碍的失眠，针灸治疗以头部局部取穴为主，配合远端取穴；以入睡、觉醒、深睡眠质量为主要障碍的失眠，针灸治疗以远端及背部取穴为主。

针对特殊类型的失眠，可在上述治疗的基础上配合特殊疗法进行治疗。

2　主要推荐意见

推荐意见	推荐级别
（1）在改善失眠患者整体睡眠质量，尤其是日间觉醒状态方面，应使用结合脏腑辨证的毫针刺法	强推荐
（2）在改善失眠患者睡眠时间和睡眠质量方面，可使用耳穴压丸疗法。其中，慢性失眠可将其作为毫针刺法的补充疗法，急性或亚急性失眠建议单独使用	弱推荐
（3）伴有日间功能障碍的失眠患者，可使用以头部安神腧穴透刺法为主，兼顾脏腑辨证的毫针刺法	弱推荐
（4）在改善入睡困难、觉醒问题及深睡眠缺少方面，可使用跷脉补泻法，身体虚弱及惧怕针刺的失眠患者建议使用本法	弱推荐
（5）在改善失眠患者入睡困难方面，可使用膀胱经及督脉皮肤针疗法，也可作为毫针刺法的配合疗法	弱推荐
（6）顽固性失眠可配合使用维生素 B_{12} 注射液穴位注射	弱推荐

简　介

《循证针灸临床实践指南：失眠》（以下简称《指南》）简介如下：

1　本《指南》制定的目标

本《指南》制定的目标是为临床医生提供治疗失眠的高质量的实用性强的针灸方案。

2　本《指南》制定的目的

本《指南》制定的目的是促进国内失眠针灸治疗方案的规范化，为临床医生提供针灸治疗失眠的可靠性证据，以确保治疗的有效性及安全性。

3　本《指南》的适用人群

本《指南》的适用人群主要为国内各级医院针灸科、神经内科、精神科医生及护理人员，针灸专业的教师及学生，针灸相关的科研工作者。

4　本《指南》适用的疾病范围

本《指南》适用于非器质性睡眠障碍的失眠症（又称原发性失眠）。老年性失眠、更年期失眠、青少年失眠可参考使用。

概　述

1　定义

1.1　西医

失眠是指对睡眠质量的不满意状况。其症状包括难以入睡、睡眠不深、易醒、多梦、早醒、醒后不易再睡、醒后不适感、疲乏或白天困倦等，容易引发焦虑、抑郁或恐惧心理，导致精神活动效率下降，妨碍社会功能[1]。

1.2　中医

失眠在中医学中称"不寐"，是指入睡困难，或睡而不酣，或时睡时醒，或醒后不能再睡，或整夜不能入睡的一类病症[2]。本病在中医古籍中还被称为"不得眠""不能眠""无眠""少睡""少寐""不眠""不睡"等，另外，该病还包括了"不得卧"及"目不瞑"中的部分内容。

2　发病率及人群分布情况

流行病学调查显示，失眠在成年人中的患病率为30%左右[3-4]。WHO全球睡眠中国区调查结果显示，中国人失眠的患病率大约为21.5%，且有日益上升的趋势[5]。该病在女性（尤其是少数民族女性）及老年人高发，处于失业或孤独状态、社会经济地位较低、正在进行药物治疗者（尤其是药物滥用或精神紊乱）发病率也偏高[6]，其他危险因素还包括共患疾病、精神异常、熬夜、轮班等[7-9]。

临床特点

根据《中国精神疾病分类与诊断标准》（CCMD－3），失眠根据持续时间不同，可分为暂时性失眠、短期失眠和慢性失眠；根据发生时间不同，可分为开始性失眠、维持性失眠、早醒或通宵不眠。虽然分类不同，但其主要临床特点基本一致。

1 病史

长期的精神压力、负面情绪、噪声等不利环境刺激。

不规律的作息时间。

反复发作的短期失眠病史。

周围存在严重的失眠症患者。

失眠家族史。

2 症状及体征

2.1 症状

本病表现为难以入睡、睡眠不深、易醒、多梦、早醒、醒后不易再睡、醒后不适感、疲乏或白天困倦等。不同类型的失眠，临床症状各有侧重。

2.1.1 开始性失眠

即入睡困难，表现为睡眠潜伏期明显延长，入睡时间一般长于30分钟。

2.1.2 维持性失眠

即睡眠浅、容易觉醒或频繁觉醒。表现为每晚要觉醒15%～20%的睡眠时间，而正常人一般不超过5%。

2.1.3 早醒

即比平时醒得早，而且常常醒后不能再入睡。

2.1.4 通宵不眠

即整个晚上不能入睡。

2.2 体征

因人而异，多数患者不伴有明显的体征，有高血压、冠心病等基础疾病的患者会出现血压升高、心悸、心前区不适等体征。

诊断标准

1 西医诊断标准及分型

1.1 诊断标准

《国际疾病分类精神疾病临床描述与诊断要点》（ICD - 10）[10] 中，非器质性失眠症（F51.0）的诊断标准如下：

主诉或是入睡困难，或是难以维持睡眠，或是睡眠质量差。

这种睡眠紊乱每周至少发生 3 次并持续 1 个月以上。

日夜专注于失眠，过分担心失眠的后果。

睡眠量和（或）质的不满意引起了明显的苦恼或影响了社会职业功能。

1.2 分型标准

2012 版《中国成人失眠诊断与治疗指南》[11] 中，失眠的临床分型标准如下：

1.2.1 急性失眠

病程小于 1 个月。

1.2.2 亚急性失眠

病程介于 1 个月到 6 个月之间。

1.2.3 慢性失眠

病程超过 6 个月。

2 中医诊断标准及分型

根据 1994 年国家中医药管理局制定的《中医病证诊断疗效标准》中"失眠诊断依据"，确定失眠的中医诊断标准及分型标准。

2.1 诊断标准

轻者入寐困难或寐而易醒，醒后不寐，重者彻夜难眠。

常伴有头痛、头昏、心悸、健忘、多梦等症状。

经实验室检查未发现异常。

2.2 分型标准

2.2.1 肝郁化火型

主症：心烦不能入睡，烦躁易怒，胸闷胁痛，目赤，口苦。

次症：头痛面红，便秘，尿黄，舌红，苔黄，脉弦数。

2.2.2 痰热内扰型

主症：睡眠不安，心烦懊恼，胸闷脘痞，口苦痰多。

次症：头晕目眩，舌红，苔黄腻，脉滑或滑数。

2.2.3 阴虚火旺型

主症：心烦不寐，或时寐时醒，手足心热，颧红潮热，口干少津。

次症：头晕耳鸣，健忘，心悸，舌红，苔少，脉细数。

2.2.4 心脾两虚型

主症：多梦易醒，或朦胧不实，心悸，健忘，神疲乏力。

次症：头晕目眩，面色不华，舌淡，苔薄，脉细弱。

2.2.5 心虚胆怯型

主症：多梦易惊，心悸，胆怯。

次症：舌淡，苔薄，脉弦细。

针灸治疗概况

针灸疗法是目前治疗失眠的非药物疗法中使用最广泛、研究最多的一种疗法，因其不良反应少、疗效可靠、不存在药物依赖和戒断反应等优点而被广泛接受。但是，由于针灸疗法本身内涵的广大性及临床应用的多样性等原因，目前研究中出现的治疗方法多种多样，总结起来，可以分为单一疗法和综合疗法两个方面。

1　现代文献

1.1　单一疗法

常用方法包括毫针刺法、电针疗法、耳穴压丸疗法、灸法、穴位注射疗法、梅花针疗法等，基础疗法为毫针刺法。

在毫针刺法的应用中，脏腑辨证是最基本的取穴方法[12]，但也有使用"镇静安神"法[13-15]、头部穴[16]、任督二脉取穴[17]、背俞穴[18]、原穴[19]、俞募配穴[20]以及子午流注[21]等按时开穴方法治疗的研究。耳穴压丸疗法比较单一，取穴多为主穴加随症取穴。灸法也可产生较好的疗效，但考虑到临床操作的安全性、简便性等问题，临床应用并不广泛，可以建议患者作为日常辅助治疗手段。穴位注射疗法主要应用于顽固性失眠，选取的腧穴多以头颈部腧穴为主[22-23]，也有选用耳穴[24]者。皮肤针疗法刺激较轻，患者接受度好，但同时因为刺激量小的问题，一般只作为辅助疗法或者作为轻症患者的治疗手段。另外，近年出现的滚刺疗法[25]实际上是皮肤针疗法的延伸，临床疗效与皮肤针疗法相当，但因为临床使用不普及，在方案中不予推荐。

除此之外，拔罐、放血、蜂针、皮内针、腕踝针、温针、穴位贴敷等，在治疗失眠方面也有一定的应用。但是，这些方法或者仅局限于某一种类型的失眠（如放血疗法用于瘀血型失眠[26]，温针疗法用于虚寒型失眠[27]），或方法比较特殊，使用时需要格外注意（如蜂针、皮内针[28]），临床使用有一定的局限性。

1.2　综合疗法

1.2.1　针刺综合疗法

主要为针刺与中药、耳穴、推拿及心理疗法的结合使用，此外，还有与放血、皮肤针、松弛疗法、穴位贴敷等方法的结合应用，但报道较少，疗效难以判定。

1.2.2　耳穴综合疗法

包括耳穴压丸与中药、推拿的结合应用，以及与灸法、穴位贴敷疗法、拔罐疗法、心理疗法、运动疗法等的联合应用，报道较少，疗效亦不确切。

1.2.3　艾灸综合疗法

这一综合疗法主要针对的是辨证中偏虚人群。配合使用的其他方法比较多，有推拿疗法、心理疗法、穴位贴敷疗法、穴位注射疗法等，据报道，疗效比较稳定。但是，因其针对的人群比较局限，疗效推广度欠佳。

1.2.4　梅花针综合疗法

与梅花针同时应用的疗法包括刮痧、拔罐、TDP照射、穴位注射、捏脊等，但是，由于此综合疗法的刺激量比较小，临床应用的局限性较大。

此外，还有关于推拿与拔罐联合使用、放血与中药联合使用、推拿与穴位注射联合应用、刮痧与心理疏导联合应用等的零散报道，因为研究极少，文献质量不高，故疗效尚不明确。

2　古代文献

古代文献中关于针灸治疗失眠的记载以单穴处方为主，另外少部分为穴组。其内容以腧穴主治、刺灸方法为主，几乎没有涉及辨证施治的内容。在选穴上，以神庭等安神穴和三阴交、太渊等远端穴较为常用；在治疗方法上，以毫针刺法最为常用，其次为灸法。

3 名医经验

近现代名医经验与现代文献相近，以毫针刺法为基本疗法。选穴上，以局部安神穴和远端穴为主穴，根据脏腑辨证选择配穴。根据患者病情可以适当选用电针疗法。除毫针刺法外，其他常用的疗法包括耳穴压丸疗法、皮肤针疗法、放血疗法等。

针灸治疗和推荐方案

1 针灸治疗的原则和特点

1.1 针灸治疗原则

针灸治疗失眠应在脏腑辨证的基础上，按患者主诉症状进行针对性治疗。以整体睡眠质量、睡眠时间、日间觉醒状态为主要障碍的失眠，针灸治疗以头部局部取穴为主，配合远端取穴；以入睡、觉醒、深睡眠质量为主要障碍的失眠，针灸治疗以远端及背部取穴为主。

针对特殊类型失眠，可在上述治疗的基础上配合特殊疗法进行治疗。

1.2 针灸治疗特点

1.2.1 临床分类的不明确性

失眠目前主要的分类方法是根据病程的长短分为急性、亚急性和慢性失眠，此分类对临床治疗尤其是针灸临床治疗失眠的参考意义不大。而如病因、人群、病情严重程度等其他分类方法，标准也并不明确，因此，依据这些标准来选择针灸治疗方案并不可行。考虑到针灸治疗失眠的临床实际，从患者主诉症状及辨证角度出发来选择相应的针灸治疗方案是比较可行的方法。

1.2.2 治疗手段的多样性

目前针灸治疗失眠的手段很多，常用的就有毫针刺法、耳穴压丸疗法、头针疗法、梅花针疗法、挑刺放血疗法、穴位注射疗法、灸法、穴位埋线疗法、火针疗法、拔罐疗法、刮痧疗法等。毫针刺法中，根据选穴方法及针刺手法的不同，又包含了跷脉补泻、头穴透刺法、腹针法、安神针法、子午流注法等许多不同的方法，这些方法虽然都能改善患者的整体睡眠质量，但事实上，每一种疗法在疗效方面都是有所侧重的。

1.2.3 疗法与主诉的对应性

失眠患者除了主诉整体睡眠质量下降外，往往还表现出在某一方面格外突出的睡眠问题，包括睡眠质量、入睡时间、睡眠时间、睡眠效率、睡眠障碍、日间功能障碍等。针灸不仅能够有效改善患者的整体睡眠质量，而且能够针对性地解决单项睡眠问题，例如，头穴透刺对于日间功能障碍可以产生针对性疗效，皮肤针疗法可以有效地改善患者入睡困难的问题等。当然，这种针对性在有些疗法中不甚明确，例如，毫针刺法虽然对日间觉醒状态有明确的疗效，但它对失眠患者的整体睡眠质量都有明显的提升，因此，在选择治疗方案时，还是应当根据患者的实际情况选择其中一种或几种方案进行治疗。

1.2.4 介入时机的重要性

介入时机对针灸治疗失眠的疗效影响较大，原则上应当是治疗时间尽量接近夜间就寝时间，但限于就诊条件，这一要求很难达到，此种情况下建议患者尽量下午进行治疗。如果患者只能上午就诊，则建议针灸治疗后午休时间不宜过长，以半小时到一小时为宜。

从病程来说，一般急性、亚急性失眠建议每天治疗一次，慢性失眠则建议隔日治疗一次，但具体治疗频率也需要参考不同疗法本身的特点。

2 主要结局指标

目前，西医评价失眠疗效的公认结局指标是以评价睡眠质量总体状况为主的各种量表，其中应用较多的是匹兹堡睡眠质量指数（PSQI）[29-30]和阿森斯睡眠量表（AIS）[29,31]；另外，也有以睡眠时间比来评价睡眠状况者，应用较多的是睡眠率[32-33]。故此三者可作为关键的结局指标。

在失眠针灸治疗的相关研究中，疗效多以有效率或痊愈率来评价，虽然有关标准多不统一，但近期研究多能根据《中医病证诊断疗效标准》中失眠的疗效评价标准来界定痊愈、有效、无效，故以此为标准的无效率可作为主要的结局指标。另外，睡眠状况自评量表、Epworth 评分、失眠患者症状积分、起效时间、疗程及复发率虽然应用相对较少，但能较全面地评价睡眠质量，因此也可作为主要结局指标。

由此可见，目前评价失眠的结局指标均以评价整体睡眠情况为主，虽然部分量表有针对睡眠质量、睡眠时间、觉醒状态等的分类分析，但就临床研究来看，大多数研究仍将关注点放在整体睡眠质量上，因此，本《指南》将评价整体睡眠质量的指标作为关键结局指标和主要结局指标。

3 注意事项

失眠患者大多较敏感且伴有情绪焦虑或抑郁，针刺时手法宜轻柔，尤其配合电针使用时，电针的刺激强度不宜过强，以患者感觉舒适为佳。

针灸治疗失眠时需要适当配合健康教育和心理疏导治疗。

针灸治疗失眠常取头面部、腕踝关节等血管较丰富位置的腧穴，容易造成皮下血肿，影响关节功能及美观，所以操作须轻柔，起针时适当延长针孔按压时间。

使用皮肤针叩刺、穴位注射疗法时，针孔局部当天避水，不宜热敷。

使用耳穴压丸疗法时，睡前半小时内不宜按压，容易兴奋皮层，增加睡眠难度。

4 健康教育和患者自我护理

4.1 健康教育

对患者的健康教育在失眠治疗中有着十分重要的临床意义，健康教育的内容一般包括：掌握睡眠知识，找出失眠原因，评估睡眠质量，合理服用药物和学会放松自己。

4.2 患者自我护理

掌握一定的睡眠知识和正确评估自我睡眠质量，可以正确认识自己的睡眠状态，有效缓解心理压力和焦虑情绪，从而有利于失眠的治疗。

找出失眠原因和合理服用药物是去除对失眠的不利因素的有效手段，尽量以非治疗方式缓解失眠问题。

放松自我的方式有很多，例如，自我按摩、睡前沐浴、泡脚等习惯，可以有效放松肌肉。

营造舒适的睡眠环境，适当欣赏轻柔音乐以放松精神。

正确评价自己，客观评价别人，保持乐观、轻松、健康的心理状态。

作息时间规律。

养成好的助眠习惯，解除睡前过量饮食、工作等不良习惯等。

5 推荐方案

5.1 毫针刺法

毫针刺法以改善全身气血状态为主要作用，因此在改善失眠患者的整体睡眠质量方面（包括睡眠质量、入睡时间、睡眠时间、睡眠效率、睡眠障碍、催眠药物应用、日间功能障碍）效果显著，尤其在改善患者日间觉醒状态方面疗效突出。研究表明，毫针刺法的疗效可优于某些西药[34-37]，也可达到与中草药相当[38]的效果。

取穴（均双侧取穴）：①主穴：神门、四神聪、三阴交。②配穴：风池、太阳、本神。

辨证：肝郁化火型配太冲、肝俞、行间；痰热内扰型配太冲、足三里；阴虚火旺型配心俞、肾俞、太溪、郄门；心脾两虚型配心俞、脾俞；心虚胆怯型配心俞、胆俞、丘墟。

操作方法：四神聪平刺，针尖方向朝向百会；本神向后平刺。其余腧穴均采用常规刺法。针刺得气后，主、配穴均使用平补平泻法，根据证型辨证取穴，行相应的补泻手法，行针 1 分钟后留针。

疗程：每次留针 30 分钟，每周 5 次，10 次为 1 个疗程，疗程之间间隔 3 天。

注意事项：临床应用时可于主穴适当配合使用电针（疏波）。

『推荐』

> 推荐建议：在改善失眠患者整体睡眠质量，尤其是日间觉醒状态方面，应使用结合脏腑辨证的毫针刺法。[GRADE 1B]

解释：针对本方案，共有相关支撑文献57篇[40-96]，经综合分析，形成证据体发现，局部安神穴与脏腑辨证结合可以有效提高患者的整体睡眠质量，且在改善其日间觉醒状态方面疗效突出。本方案支撑证据数量较大，偏倚风险较低，经GRADE评价、专家共识后，因其文献设计质量、一致性及精确性高，最终证据体质量等级为中。

5.2 耳穴压丸疗法

耳穴压丸疗法能够平衡大脑皮层的兴奋与抑制，从而使大脑皮层的功能活动趋于正常。因此，其疗效主要体现在改善患者的睡眠时间、睡眠质量方面，其对于睡眠其他方面的改善尚少有研究。另外，在失眠治疗中，毫针刺法结束后采用耳穴压丸的方式，在补充针灸治疗的基础上，更能给予大脑皮层持久的小剂量刺激，更符合失眠的疾病特点。

取穴：①主穴：神门、皮质下、交感、内分泌、枕。②配穴：心、肾。

辨证：肝郁化火型配肝、胆；阴虚火旺型配肾、肝；心脾两虚型配脾、心、胃；心虚胆怯型配心、胆。

操作方法：针刺结束后，将王不留行籽（或磁珠）贴于0.5cm×0.5cm的医用胶布中央，耳穴常规消毒后，将粘有王不留行籽（或磁珠）的胶布贴在上述耳穴，并适度按压，使耳穴有胀、热、微痛感。每晚睡前按1次，约5分钟，以耳郭微红、微热为度，隔天换贴1次，双耳交替。

疗程：常规针灸治疗后进行，每3天更换1次，4次为1个疗程。

注意事项：①耳穴压丸疗法一般作为毫针刺法的延续治疗方法，单独使用疗效有限；只有短期或者轻度失眠患者单独使用可获较满意的疗效。②如果耳穴按压后疼痛较剧烈，睡前可将其除去，防止因疼痛而影响睡眠。

『推荐』

> 推荐建议：在改善失眠患者睡眠时间和睡眠质量方面，可使用耳穴压丸疗法。其中，慢性失眠可将其作为毫针刺法的补充疗法；急性或亚急性失眠建议单独使用。[GRADE 2C]

解释：针对本方案，共有相关支撑文献8篇[97-104]，经综合分析，形成证据体发现，通过对相应耳穴的刺激来平衡大脑皮层的兴奋与抑制作用，对于改善失眠患者的睡眠时间、睡眠质量有较好的临床疗效。本方案形成时间较短，缺乏古代证据支撑，且证据数量不多，偏倚风险相对较高，但此方案有众多的现代医家经验支撑，因此经GRADE评价、专家共识后，因其文献设计质量、一致性、精确性不高，但专家经验支撑力强，最终证据体质量等级为低。

5.3 头穴透刺法

透刺法作为平刺或斜刺的延伸应用，是通经行气、增强刺激的一种重要手法。将其应用于头部腧穴，在增强腧穴本身的镇静安神作用的同时，可以有效疏通头部郁阻的经脉，因此更适用于伴有日间功能障碍的失眠患者，在改善其睡眠时间和睡眠质量的同时，可以有效提高日间活动效率。相关研究表明其疗效优于毫针刺法[39]。

取穴：①主穴：前神聪透神庭、左右头临泣透左右神聪、后神聪透强间。②配穴：络却透通天、承光透曲差。

操作方法：由前神聪进针，平刺透向神庭；由头临泣进针，平刺透向同侧神聪；由后神聪进针，平刺透向强间。采用直径0.35~0.40mm、长度40~50mm的毫针，针身与头皮呈15°角，快速刺入头皮下，当针尖到达帽状腱膜下层，指下感到阻力减小时，将针与头皮平行，继续捻转进针，各穴进针深度为 1～1.5 寸，然后快速小幅度左右捻针，每穴行针约 1 分钟，取得较强针感后留针。

疗程：每次留针 30 分钟，每天 1 次，5 次为 1 个疗程，疗程之间间隔 2 天。

注意事项：临床应用时，头穴透刺作为主要治疗方法，需同时根据患者病情，辨证加用其他腧穴，针刺方法采用常规刺法。

『推荐』

> 推荐建议：伴有日间功能障碍的失眠患者，可使用以头部安神腧穴透刺法为主，兼顾脏腑辨证的毫针刺法。[GRADE 2C]

解释：针对本方案，共有相关支撑文献 3 篇[105-107]，经综合分析，形成证据体发现，通过对头部局部腧穴进行透刺，不仅能够加强镇静安神的作用，而且能够增加其疏通头部经气的功效，对于伴有日间功能障碍的失眠患者更加适用。本方案虽然支撑证据少，但存在质量相对较高的证据[11]，同时在专家共识阶段也得到专家的一致支持，因此经 GRADE 评价、专家共识后，因其文献设计质量较高，一致性、精确性不高，但专家经验支撑力较高，最终证据体质量等级为低。

5.4 跷脉补泻法

由于人体的睡眠与阴阳跷脉的平衡有密切的关系，因此，泻阳跷、补阴跷，使得阴阳达到平衡，就成为了一种重要的治疗方法。其中，泻阳跷（申脉）可以有效改善觉醒时间、觉醒次数和深睡眠状况，而补阴跷（照海）则可以有效改善入睡困难的情况，二者侧重点有异。跷脉补泻法为泻阳跷和补阴跷的结合运用，在实际应用中需要根据患者病情的不同，酌情使用。

取穴：申脉、照海。

操作方法：患者仰卧位，针具、腧穴常规消毒后，先针照海，行捻转补法；再针申脉，行捻转泻法。

疗程：每次留针 30 分钟，每天 1 次，10 次为 1 个疗程，疗程之间间隔 3 天。

注意事项：①此法需在明辨阴阳侧重的基础上灵活使用，且通常可与毫针刺法合用。②此法中的两穴在针刺时容易有放电感出现，从而增加患者的紧张心理，因此在治疗前需要做好相应的告知和解释工作。③此法用穴少，身体虚弱及惧怕针刺者可考虑使用。

『推荐』

> 推荐建议：在改善入睡困难、觉醒问题及深睡眠缺少方面，可使用跷脉补泻法。身体虚弱及惧怕针刺的失眠患者建议使用本法。[GRADE 2D]

解释：针对本方案，共有相关支撑文献 7 篇[108-114]，经综合分析，形成证据体发现，本方案通过泻阳跷、补阴跷，能够达到平衡阴阳的作用，从而可以针对性地改善患者入睡困难、觉醒问题、深睡眠缺少等问题。本方案证据数量不多，且 GRADE 评价级别极低，虽然专家共识一致性较高，可以对方案进行推荐，但无法提高其证据级别，因此，本方案最终证据体质量等级为极低。

5.5 皮肤针疗法

运用皮肤针疗法治疗失眠，主要通过刺激膀胱经第一、二侧线及督脉来达到调整脏腑的功能，疏达任、督脉气，除了能有效改善睡眠质量外，还能有效缩短患者的入睡时间。研究表明，本疗法单独使用时可达到与某些西药相当的疗效[36]。此疗法的突出优势在于不易产生耐药性及不良反应。

取穴：背部足太阳膀胱经第一、二侧线及督脉。

操作方法：患者俯卧位，用皮肤针沿膀胱经第一、二侧线由上向下，督脉由下向上进行叩击，每次叩击之间的距离为 0.5cm，反复叩击 5 分钟，以皮肤潮红为度。膀胱经第一、二侧线实证可叩至皮肤微出血。

疗程：每次治疗 15～20 分钟，隔天 1 次，10 次为 1 个疗程。

注意事项：①此疗法可单独使用，也可作为毫针刺法的配合疗法。②如叩刺出血，嘱患者24小时针孔避水，防止感染。

『推荐』

> 推荐建议：在改善失眠患者入睡困难方面，可使用膀胱经及督脉皮肤针疗法；此法也可作为毫针刺法的配合疗法。[GRADE 2D]

解释：针对本方案，共有相关支撑文献8篇[115-122]，经综合分析，形成证据体发现，通过对膀胱经、督脉的皮部进行刺激，不仅能够调整相应脏腑的功能，更能有效调顺督脉经气，从而改善患者的睡眠质量，尤其是解决入睡困难的问题。本方案证据数量不多，偏倚风险较高，GRADE评价级别为极低，虽然有专家经验证据支持，且专家共识一致性较高，可以对方案进行推荐，但无法提高其证据级别，因此，本方案最终证据体质量等级为极低。

5.6 穴位注射疗法

穴位注射疗法将针刺作用、药理作用、药水对腧穴的渗透刺激作用结合在一起发挥综合效果，对于某些顽固性疾病效果可靠。主要用作顽固性失眠的辅助疗法。但目前尚无有力证据证明其与其他疗法在疗效方面的优劣关系。

取穴：风池、心俞。

药物：维生素 B_{12} 注射液。

操作方法：在上述腧穴注射，局部出现酸、麻、胀或放射感后，回抽，如无回血则可缓慢注入维生素 B_{12} 注射液，每穴0.1mg。左、右穴交替进行。

疗程：每天1次，10次为1个疗程。

注意事项：①穴位注射当天局部避水，避免热敷。②注射局部吸收不良时，可待吸收完全后再行治疗。

『推荐』

> 推荐建议：顽固性失眠可配合使用维生素 B_{12} 注射液穴位注射疗法。[GRADE 2D]

解释：针对本方案，共有相关支撑文献21篇[123-143]，经综合分析，形成证据体发现，穴位注射疗法通过综合腧穴、药物等的作用，对于顽固性失眠可以产生较好的治疗效果，因此可以作为顽固性失眠的辅助治疗方法。本方案证据数量虽然较多，但偏倚风险较高，GRADE评价级别为极低，虽然有一定数量的专家共识，但无法提高其证据级别，因此，本方案最终证据体质量等级为极低。

参考文献

[1] 中华医学会精神科分会．中国精神障碍分类与诊断标准［M］．第3版．济南：山东科学技术出版社，2001．

[2] 中华中医药学会．中医内科常见病诊疗指南［M］．北京：中国中医药出版社，2008．

[3] Thomas Roth, Insomnia：Definition, Prevalence, Etiology, and Consequences［J］．Clin Sleep Med, 2007, 3（5）：7－10．

[4] Ohayon MM. Prevalence of DSM－IV diagnostic criteria of insomnia：distinguishing insomnia related to mental disorders from sleep disorders［J］．J Psychiatr Res, 1997, 31：333－346．

[5] 赵晖．针灸治疗失眠的临床研究概况［J］．湖北中医杂志，2008，30（7）：60－62．

[6] Mellinger GD, Balter MB, Uhlenhuth EH. Insomnia and its treatment：Prevalence and correlates［J］．Arch Gen Psychiatry, 2001, 42：225－232．

[7] Katz DA, McHorney CA. Clinical correlates of insomnia in patients with chronic illness［J］．Arch Intern Med, 1998, 158：1099－1107．

[8] Ford DE, Kamerow DB. Epidemiologic study of sleep disturbances and psychiatric disorders［J］．An opportunity for prevention, 1989, 262：1479－1484．

[9] Roth T, Roehrs T. Insomnia：epidemiology, characteristics, and consequences［J］．Clin Cornerstone, 2003, 5：5－15．

[10] 世界卫生组织．范肖冬译．精神与行为障碍分类临床描述与诊断要点［M］．第10版．北京：人民卫生出版社，1993．

[11] 中华医学会神经病学分会睡眠障碍学组．中国成人失眠诊断与治疗指南［J］．中华神经科杂志，2012，45（7）：534．

[12] 沈兴城．针刺治疗失眠［J］．中国临床医学研究杂志，2004，113：11879－11880．

[13] 张欣，严兴科，唐强．镇静安神针法与针刺跷脉法治疗失眠的临床疗效比较［J］．时珍国医国药，2010，21（3）：686－687．

[14] 张欣，严兴科，王富春．镇静安神针法与针刺经外奇穴法治疗失眠的临床研究［J］．南京中医药大学学报，2010，26（1）：24－26．

[15] 张欣，严兴科，王国松．镇静安神针法与针刺背俞穴法治疗失眠的临床疗效比较［J］．环球中医药，2009，2（2）：127－129．

[16] 曹仁俊，石青．电针头部奇穴为主治疗不寐30例［J］．按摩与导引，2001，17（2）：20．

[17] 胡雨华，李国．针刺调理任督二脉治疗失眠症40例［J］．陕西中医，2009，30（11）：1519－1520．

[18] 周艳丽，杜彩霞，高希言．针刺调理五脏背俞穴治疗失眠症40例［J］．中医研究，2009，22（4）：56－57．

[19] 常伟．原穴为主针灸治验不寐证328例［J］．中国民间疗法，2009，17（6）：6－7．

[20] 黄峥．俞募配穴法治疗顽固性失眠2例［J］．安徽中医学院学报，1997，16（4）：49－50．

[21] 杨梅，刘芳，段晓蓉．子午流注针法治疗失眠症疗效观察［J］．安徽中医临床杂志，2003，15（4）：321－322．

[22] 李金明，刘芳．安眠穴穴位注射治疗失眠38例［J］．中国针灸，2004，24（11）：749．

[23] 邹娴，李爱云．穴位注射治疗不寐的疗效观察［J］．实用中西医结合临床，2010，10

（2）：58.

[24] 冯桂林．丹参液耳穴注射治疗失眠症 50 例［J］．内蒙古中医药，1994，（1）：20.

[25] 罗玲，胡幼平，余曙光，等．滚针治疗失眠症临床疗效研究［J］．中国针灸，2006，26（3）：183－185.

[26] 吴超，戴衍．三棱针刺血络治疗失眠［J］．中国康复，2004，19（2）：118.

[27] 范郁山，姚春．温针灸法治疗失眠 37 例［J］．陕西中医，2003，24（2）：164.

[28] 王长来．皮内针治疗失眠 210 例疗效观察［J］．成都医药，1997，23（3）：183.

[29] 何凤麟．平调阴阳针刺法治疗顽固性失眠临床观察［J］．中国中医急症，2010，19（6）：940－941.

[30] 翁明．电针治疗老年性失眠疗效量表分析［J］．针灸临床杂志，2007，23（5）：33－34.

[31] 罗仁瀚．针刺治疗失眠症的临床研究［J］．针灸临床杂志，2008，24（12）：5－6.

[32] 严兴科．"镇静安神"针法对心脾两虚型失眠患者匹兹堡睡眠指数的影响［J］．针刺研究，2010，35（3）：222－225.

[33] 曾宪锋．针刺治疗失眠 80 例疗效观察［J］．针灸临床杂志，2005，21（12）：22.

[34] 柴路．经络针刺结合耳针治疗失眠 40 例［J］．光明中医，2010，25（5）：821－822.

[35] 侯春英．针刺治疗失眠 150 例疗效观察［J］．新中医，2005，37（3）：61－62.

[36] 王成伟．滚针对非器质性慢性失眠症患者生活质量的影响：随机对照研究［J］．中国针灸，2006，26（7）：461－465.

[37] 岳宝安．针刺五心穴治疗顽固性失眠 30 例［J］．陕西中医，2009，30（8）：1045－1046.

[38] 吕晃祯．刺血配以电针治疗肝郁化火型失眠症的临床观察［D］．广州中医药大学硕士学位论文，2010.

[39] 董建萍．头部透穴法治疗失眠症随机对照观察［J］．中国针灸，2008，28（3）：159－162.

[40] 柴路．经络针刺结合耳针治疗失眠 40 例［J］．光明中医，2010，25（5）：821－822.

[41] 吕晃祯．刺血配以电针治疗肝郁化火型失眠症的临床观察［D］．广州中医药大学硕士学位论文，2010.

[42] 侯春英．针刺治疗失眠 150 例疗效观察［J］．新中医，2005，37（3）：61－62.

[43] 岳宝安．针刺五心穴治疗顽固性失眠 30 例［J］．陕西中医，2009，30（8）：1045－1046.

[44] 何凤麟．平调阴阳针刺法治疗顽固性失眠临床观察［J］．中国中医急症，2010，19（6）：940.

[45] 翁明．电针治疗老年性失眠疗效量表分析［J］．针灸临床杂志，2007，23（5）：33－34.

[46] 刘建武．"调阴阳五脏"针法治疗失眠的临床及实验研究［D］．广州中医药大学硕士学位论文，2006.

[47] 王麟鹏．针刺对原发性失眠患者日间觉醒状态的影响［D］．第 2 届中国睡眠医学论坛论文汇编，2007.

[48] 郭静．针刺对原发性失眠患者日间觉醒状态的影响［J］．北京中医药，2008，27（7）：497－499.

[49] 任珊．针刺治疗失眠选穴优化方案的临床研究［J］．中医学报，2009，24（6）：46－47.

[50] 任珊．针刺治疗失眠选穴组方筛选的临床研究［D］．2010 年中国针灸学会脑病专业委员会、中国针灸学会循证针灸专业委员会学术大会论文集，2010.

[51] 董锐．以督脉和任脉为主针灸治疗失眠 12 例［J］．中医外治杂志，2011，20（1）：36－37.

[52] 张欣．针刺疗法治疗失眠的优选方案及疗效评价的临床研究和机理探讨［D］．黑龙江中医药大学硕士学位论文，2009.

［53］ 尹红博．针刺阴阳跷脉之申脉、照海穴治疗原发性失眠的临床研究［D］．山东中医药大学硕士学位论文，2008．

［54］ 王盛春．电针神门、四神聪对原发性失眠患者多导睡眠图的影响［J］．山东医药，2010，50（41）：13－15．

［55］ 寇吉友．调脏安神法针刺治疗失眠的临床研究［D］．黑龙江中医药大学硕士学位论文，2003．

［56］ 伟杰．针刺跷脉穴治疗失眠的临床研究［J］．中华中医药学刊，2011，29（2）：413－414．

［57］ 蔡炼．从脾胃论治失眠的针刺临床研究［D］．北京中医药大学硕士学位论文，2006．

［58］ 陈俊如．电针四关穴为主治疗肝郁化火型失眠症的临床研究［D］．广州中医药大学硕士学位论文，2010．

［59］ 大前．针刺督脉经腧穴为主治疗心肾不交型失眠症的临床疗效观察［D］．南京中医药大学硕士学位论文，2009．

［60］ 韩纪琴．针灸治疗心脾两虚型失眠症30例疗效观察［J］．山西中医学院学报，2010，11（5）：36－37．

［61］ 罗文政．解郁调神针刺法治疗失眠伴抑郁障碍疗效观察［J］．中国针灸，2010，30（11）：899－903．

［62］ 吕柏欣．电针百会、印堂穴治疗单纯性失眠的临床研究［D］．广州中医药大学硕士学位论文，2009．

［63］ 吕锦春．针刺治疗原发性睡眠障碍的临床观察［J］．中国现代医生，2010，48（29）：42－43．

［64］ 毛亮．针刺治疗心脾两虚型失眠的临床观察［D］．辽宁中医药大学硕士学位论文，2009．

［65］ 彭冬青．电针风池穴治疗失眠症临床观察［J］．中国中医药现代远程教育，2008，6（12）：1492－1493．

［66］ 齐丽珍．项丛刺治疗失眠症76例疗效观察［D］．中国针灸学会第八届全国中青年针灸推拿学术研讨会论文汇编，2008．

［67］ 齐丽珍．项丛刺治疗失眠症疗效观察［J］．中国针灸，2008，28（12）：861－864．

［68］ 陶红星．针刺经外奇穴治疗失眠症58例临床研究［J］．吉林中医药，2009，29（1）：52－53．

［69］ 严兴科．"镇静安神"针法对心脾两虚型失眠患者匹兹堡睡眠指数的影响［J］．针刺研究，2010，35（3）：222－225．

［70］ 杨自威．针刺为主治疗失眠症的临床研究［J］．上海针灸杂志，2008，27（4）：6－8．

［71］ 张金媛．针刺五脏俞为主对慢性失眠症患者睡眠质量影响的临床观察［D］．南京中医药大学硕士学位论文，2010．

［72］ 张璞璘．针刺四神聪穴治疗失眠的多中心随机对照研究［J］．中医杂志，2008，49（8）：712－714．

［73］ 张蕊．针灸治疗失眠55例［J］．陕西中医，2010，31（10）：1384－1385．

［74］ 张欣．镇静安神针法与针刺经外奇穴法治疗失眠的临床研究［J］．南京中医药大学学报，2010，26（1）：24－26．

［75］ 张欣．镇静安神针法与针刺跷脉穴法治疗失眠的PSQI指数与临床疗效比较［J］．辽宁中医杂志，2009，36（12）：2158－2159．

［76］ 张颖颖．调督健脑针刺法治疗失眠症的临床研究［J］．上海针灸杂志，2009，28（3）：140－142．

［77］ 张永乐．安神解郁针法治疗失眠症临床观察［J］．上海中医药杂志，2009，43（7）：24－25．

［78］ 张悦．从心肝论治失眠的针刺临床研究［D］．辽宁中医药大学硕士学位论文，2007．

［79］ 李娟．电针印堂、神庭穴治疗失眠症的随机对照观察［D］．广州中医药大学硕士学位论

文，2009.

［80］李新艳．针刺治疗中老年失眠症的临床研究［D］．北京中医药大学硕士学位论文，2008.

［81］李新艳．针刺治疗中老年失眠症的临床研究［J］．天津中医药，2010，27（5）：386－388.

［82］孙兆元．针刺太溪、三阴交、涌泉穴治疗老年人失眠40例［J］．陕西中医，2010，31（6）：731－732.

［83］岳公雷．镇静安神法与阴阳跷脉法治疗失眠（心脾两虚型）疗效对照研究［D］．长春中医药大学硕士学位论文，2008.

［84］张颖颖．通督调神针刺法对失眠症患者睡眠质量及心理状态影响的临床研究［D］．南京中医药大学硕士学位论文，2009.

［85］周丹．镇静安神法对心脾两虚型失眠患者脑血流状况的影响［D］．长春中医药大学硕士学位论文，2007.

［86］陈理．督脉五穴治疗失眠26例临床观察［J］．江苏中医药，2008，40（4）：53－54.

［87］吴希．针刺周氏调神方对原发性失眠患者睡眠质量影响的随机对照研究［D］．北京中医药大学硕士学位论文，2007.

［88］徐世芬．健脑调卫针刺治疗失眠的时效性临床观察［J］．河北中医，2010，32（6）：886－888.

［89］徐世芬．健脑调卫针刺治疗失眠的时效性临床观察［D］．全国第四次中医科研方法学暨花生枝叶治疗失眠症研究成果汇报学术研讨会专家讲课和学术论文集，2009.

［90］严兴科．镇静安神针法治疗失眠的临床观察［J］．时珍国医国药，2009，20（8）：2004－2005.

［91］叶仿武．调督针法对匹茨堡睡眠质量指数的影响［J］．甘肃中医，2011，24（1）：36－38.

［92］张春华．电针四神聪穴对失眠症PSG及PSQI的影响［D］．山东大学硕士学位论文，2006.

［93］王成伟．滚针对非器质性慢性失眠症患者生活质量的影响随机对照研究［J］．中国针灸，2006，26（7）：461－465.

［94］贺普仁．毫针疗法图解［M］．济南：山东科学技术出版社，1998.

［95］程莘农．中国针灸学［M］．北京：人民卫生出版社，1964.

［96］田从豁，臧俊岐．中国灸法集粹［M］．沈阳：辽宁科学技术出版社，1987.

［97］高希言．耳穴在治疗失眠中作用的临床观察［D］．第12届全国耳穴诊治学术研讨会论文汇编，2009.

［98］胡伟．耳穴埋藏对中青年失眠症患者睡眠功能的影响［J］．中国康复，2010，25（6）：450－452.

［99］胡伟．耳穴压丸对中年失眠症患者睡眠功能的影响［J］．World Journal of Acupuncture － Moxibustion，2010，20（4）：23－28.

［100］林博郎．耳穴压丸治疗失眠的临床研究［D］．北京中医药大学硕士学位论文，2007.

［101］刘卫红．耳穴压丸疗法对睡眠障碍为主的亚健康状态干预作用的研究［J］．中医药学刊，2005，23（4）：637－638.

［102］刘卫红．耳穴压丸疗法干预睡眠障碍为主的亚健康状态临床随机对照研究［J］．中国中医基础医学杂志，2008，14（3）：222－223.

［103］刘卫红．耳穴压丸疗法干预睡眠障碍为主的亚健康状态临床随机对照研究［J］．中华中医药学刊，2008，26（2）：298－299.

［104］骆晓林．耳穴压籽治疗大学生失眠症21例疗效观察［J］．中医药导报，2010，16（2）：46－47.

[105] 董建萍．头部透穴法治疗失眠症随机对照观察［J］．中国针灸，2008，28（3）：159－162.

[106] 张治强．头穴透刺法治疗失眠的临床观察［J］．光明中医，2010，25（9）：1658－1660.

[107] 周章玲．头穴透刺法治疗失眠症的随机对照研究［J］．中西医结合学报，2010，8（2）：126－130.

[108] 尹红博．针刺阴阳跷脉之申脉、照海穴治疗原发性失眠的临床研究［D］．山东中医药大学硕士学位论文，2008.

[109] 张会珍．针刺照海申脉为主治疗顽固性失眠［J］．浙江中医杂志，2005，4：169.

[110] 刘伟哲．针刺申脉、照海穴为主治疗失眠症52例［J］．World Journal of Acupuncture - Moxibustion，2007，17（2）：61－63.

[111] 马新平．针刺照海、申脉治疗肝郁化火型失眠的疗效观察［J］．四川中医，2011，29（3）：119－120.

[112] 王如杰．针刺申脉、照海治疗顽固性失眠40例临床观察［J］．四川中医，2008，26（4）：123.

[113] 王世广．针刺照海、申脉为主治疗不寐症临床观察［J］．中国针灸，2005，25（11）：771－772.

[114] 张会珍．照海、申脉为主治疗顽固性失眠临床观察［J］．四川中医，2003，21（6）：75－76.

[115] 田文海．梅花针叩刺治疗失眠50例疗效观察［D］．中国特种针法应用与针灸临床学术交流大会论文集，2000.

[116] 程建华．梅花针叩打法治疗失眠22例疗效观察［J］．中国社区医师，2006，22（1）：43.

[117] 黄立雄．梅花针治疗失眠症34例［J］．上海针灸杂志，2005，24（8）：13.

[118] 李丽娟．皮肤针疗法治疗不寐20例［J］．针灸临床杂志，2000，16（8）：32.

[119] 秦爱国．梅花针叩刺治疗不寐76例［J］．中国针灸，1996，（12）：46－47.

[120] 王红梅．梅花针叩打治疗失眠48例［J］．长春中医药大学学报，2008，24（1）：59.

[121] 庄丹红．梅花针叩刺背俞穴治疗顽固性失眠42例［J］．上海针灸杂志，2004，23（5）：33.

[122] 庄丹红．梅花针叩刺背俞穴治疗顽固性失眠42例［J］．中国针灸，2004，24（6）：428.

[123] 史玲．天麻素穴位注射治疗失眠症40例［J］．中医外治杂志，2010，19（1）：44.

[124] 邹娴．穴位注射治疗不寐的疗效观察［J］．实用中西医结合临床，2010，10（2）：52－71.

[125] 白晓莉．穴位注射治疗失眠50例疗效观察［J］．光明中医，2006，21（3）：39.

[126] 龚瑗瑗．风池穴穴位注射生理盐水治疗焦虑性失眠29例临床观察［J］．实用中西医结合临床，2010，10（1）：16－17.

[127] 李种泰．穴位注射治疗心肾不交型失眠55例［J］．辽宁中医杂志，2006，33（1）：98.

[128] 李种泰．穴位注射治疗心肾不交型失眠55例［J］．四川中医，2006，24（2）：103－104.

[129] 班旭升．穴位注射治疗顽固性失眠120例［J］．上海针灸杂志，1998，17（4）：21.

[130] 戴建林．丹参穴位注射治疗失眠症100例［J］．四川中医，1986，（4）：42.

[131] 范景宽．刺五加注射液结合针剂治疗心脾两虚型失眠96例疗效观察［J］．辽宁中医杂志，2008，35（6）：895.

[132] 冯桂林．丹参液耳穴注射治疗失眠症50例［J］．内蒙古中医药，1994：20.

[133] 李焕堂．异丙嗪穴位注射法治疗失眠［J］．临床荟萃，1990，5（2）：72.

[134] 李金明．安眠穴穴位注射治疗失眠38例［J］．中国针灸，2004，24（11）：749.

[135] 刘芳琴．穴位注射治疗顽固性失眠［J］．农村医药报，2003.

[136] 刘芳琴．穴位注射治疗顽固性失眠80例［J］．中国民间疗法，2003：19.

[137] 马延平．维生素 B_1 穴位注射治疗不寐证20例观察［J］．新疆中医药，2001，19（1）：37.

［138］孙海侠．背俞穴药物注射治疗顽固性失眠 28 例疗效观察［J］．白求恩医科大学学报，1998，24（6）：659．

［139］万静．穴位封闭治疗顽固性失眠 35 例临床观察［J］．现代康复，2001，5（8）：120．

［140］王宁生．当归注射液穴位注射治疗失眠症 50 例临床观察［J］．中西医结合杂志，1983：319．

［141］许静芳．维生素 B_{12} 穴位注射治疗不寐 134 例观察［J］．甘肃中医，2003，16（2）：36－37．

［142］杨明英．中西药穴位注射治疗失眠 52 例［J］．实用中医药杂志，1999，15（10）：17．

［143］张小兵．穴位注射治疗失眠 156 例疗效观察［J］．上海针灸杂志，2006，25（8）：9．

附　录

1　本《指南》专家组成员和编写组成员

专家组成员

姓名	性别	学历/职称	工作单位	研究方向
赵京生	男	硕士，教授	中国中医科学院针灸研究所	针灸基础理论
程海英	女	学士，主任医师	首都医科大学附属北京中医医院	针灸临床
陈　枫	男	学士，主任医师	中国中医科学院望京医院神经内科	针灸临床
王克健	男	硕士，主任医师	中国中医科学院西苑医院针灸科	针灸临床
薛　爽	女	硕士，主任医师	中日友好医院神经内科	神经内科
范为宇	女	学士，研究员	中国中医科学院信息研究所	情报信息
詹思延	女	博士，教授	北京大学公共卫生学院流行病学与卫生统计学系	循证医学

编写组成员

	姓名	性别	学历/职称	工作单位	课题中的分工
组长	杨金洪	女	学士，主任医师	中国中医科学院针灸医院	总负责人，负责课题设计并形成推荐
组员	胡　静	女	硕士，主治医师	中国中医科学院针灸医院	文献检索、文献评价
	王　兵	女	硕士，副主任医师	中国中医科学院针灸医院	文献检索
	张　宁	女	硕士，副主任医师	中国中医科学院针灸医院	文献检索
	姜爱平	女	硕士，主任医师	中国中医科学院针灸医院	文献评价
	曹建萍	女	学士，主任医师	中国中医科学院针灸医院	文献评价
	尹红红	女	学士，副主任护师	中国中医科学院针灸医院	课题管理
	杨逢春	女	学士，硕士研究生	中国中医科学院针灸研究所	电话咨询、联络、资料整理

2 临床问题

2.1 临床问卷

2.1.1 医生问卷

国家中医药管理局
失眠针灸临床实践指南意见征询稿
（医生问卷）

省/直辖市/自治区＿＿＿＿＿＿＿＿＿＿＿　　　　　职称＿＿＿＿＿＿＿＿＿

尊敬的各位针灸专家以及同行，首先感谢您在百忙之中填写这份问卷。

为了协助国家中医药管理局标准化研究项目《失眠针灸临床实践指南》的顺利进行，使得这份指南具有最大程度上的实用性和针对性，现需要就相关针灸临床问题向您征询意见，请您逐项独立填写本问卷。对于您对本项目的支持，我们再次表示衷心的感谢。

填写说明：

1. 本问卷的征询对象为针灸医师及针灸临床从业者。

2. 请结合您的临床经验独立填写本问卷。

3. 本问卷第一部分为选择及排序性问题，请在选择适当答案的基础上，按照每一问题后面的要求对该题目的相关选项进行排序（未要求的不必排序）。

4. 本问卷第二部分为选择性问题，请您在认为适当的表格内画√即可。例如，您"非常关注"失眠的"临床表现"，则只需在第3行对应"非常关注"的表格内画√；如果您还有其他意见或建议请写在表格下面相应问题的空白处。

5. 填写本问卷时请您保证字迹清楚，容易辨认。

失眠针灸临床指南课题组

2010 年

第一部分

1. 您认为针灸主要对下列哪种类型的失眠疗效可靠？
   A. 原发性失眠　①单纯性失眠　②遗传性失眠　③更年期失眠　④产后失眠
   B. 继发性失眠　①脑血管病失眠（包括脑血管硬化、脑梗死、脑外伤等引起的失眠）
   　　　　　　　②内科疾病失眠（包括肺心病、风湿、糖尿病、肢体麻木等引起的失眠）
   　　　　　　　③精神疾病失眠（包括抑郁症、焦虑症、精神分裂症等引起的失眠）
   　　　　　　　④药物依赖性失眠（主要是指长期服用安眠药，停药或者无效后出现的失眠）

   请将您的选项（如 A①）按疗效由高到低的顺序进行排序（前三项）＿＿＿＿＿＿＿

2. 您认为失眠中最常见的证型是：
   A. 心脾两虚　　　B. 气血两虚　　　C. 气阴两虚　　　D. 心胆气虚　　　E. 心肾不交
   F. 脾虚湿盛　　　G. 心肝火旺　　　H. 肝郁化火　　　I. 胃腑失和　　　J. 胆郁痰扰
   K. 其他＿＿＿＿＿＿＿＿＿＿＿＿＿＿＿＿＿＿＿

   请将您的选项按证型由常见到相对不常见顺序进行排序（前五项）＿＿＿＿＿＿＿

3. 您在治疗失眠的过程中经常使用的穴位类型有：
   A. 与"神"有关的穴（如神门、神庭、四神聪、本神等）　　　B. 背俞穴
   C. 经外奇穴　　　　　　　　　　　　　　　　　　　　　　D. 八脉交会穴
   E. 手足部特定穴　　　　　　　　　　　　　　　　　　　　F. 辨证脏腑配穴
   G. 其他＿＿＿＿＿＿＿＿＿＿＿＿＿＿＿＿＿＿＿

   请将您的选项按使用频率由高到低的顺序进行排序（前五项）＿＿＿＿＿＿＿

4. 您在治疗失眠时常用的方法有：
   A. 针刺　　　B. 艾灸　　　C. 穴位贴敷　　　D. 拔罐　　　E. 耳穴压丸　　　F. 刺络放血
   G. 电针　　　H. 头皮针　　I. 穴位注射　　　J. 梅花针　　K. 皮内针　　　L. 穴位埋线
   M. 指针　　　N. 腕踝针　　O. 腹针　　　　　P. 其他＿＿＿＿＿＿＿＿＿＿＿＿＿＿＿

   请将您的选项按使用频率由高到低的顺序进行排序（前五项）＿＿＿＿＿＿＿

5. 您认为不同类型的失眠常用的治疗方法有哪些（只需列出前五项即可）？
   （选项与第 4 题相同，可多选，对于您认为疗效不确切的类型，可以不予填写）
   （1）单纯性失眠：
   （2）遗传性失眠：
   （3）更年期失眠：
   （4）产后失眠：
   （5）脑血管病失眠：
   （6）内科疾病失眠：
   （7）精神疾病失眠：
   （8）药物依赖性失眠：

6. 在临床应用中，除了针灸治疗，您认为是否还需要配合其他疗法？如果需要，请选择：

A. 不需要

B. 需要 　　①推拿按摩 　　②足浴/足底按摩 　　③中药
　　　　　　④西药 　　　　⑤功能性仪器 　　⑥其他

请将您的选项按使用频率由高到低的顺序进行排序（只列出前五项，选 A 则不需要填写本项）
_____

7. 您认为"补泻"在针灸治疗失眠中重要吗？如果重要，常用的方法是什么？

A. 不重要 　　B. 重要 　　①泻阳补阴法 ②泻法 ③补法 ④平补平泻法 ⑤其他_____

8. 您认为针灸治疗失眠最佳的治疗时间是：

A. 15～20 分钟 　　B. 30 分钟 　　C. 40～50 分钟 　　D. 1 小时

9. 您认为针灸治疗失眠最佳的治疗频率是：

A. 1 天 2 次 　　B. 1 天 1 次 　　C. 2 天 1 次 　　D. 1 周 2 次

10. 您认为针灸治疗失眠的疗程应当是：

A. 7 次 1 疗程 　　B. 10 次 1 疗程 　　C. 14 次 1 疗程 　　D. 20 次 1 疗程

第二部分

请您根据对下面 22 个问题的关注度，在每一个问题后面适当的表格内画√。

项目	不关注 0分	一般关注 1分	关注 2分	比较关注 3分	非常关注 4分
1. 定义					
2. 临床流行病情况					
3. 临床表现					
4. 中医诊断					
5. 西医诊断					
6. 西医分型					
7. 辨证分型					
8. 危险因素/诱发因素					
9. 针灸介入时机					
10. 针灸治疗原则					
11. 针灸选穴					
12. 针灸方法及具体操作					
13. 疗程及治疗频率					
14. 疗效及预后					
15. 注意事项					
16. 不良反应					

项目	不关注 0分	一般关注 1分	关注 2分	比较关注 3分	非常关注 4分
17. 禁忌证					
18. 疗效评价方法					
19. 卫生经济学评价					
20. 推荐方案的支持证据及其级别					
21. 配合使用的其他中医方法					
22. 配合使用的西医方法					

除了上述问题，您认为该指南中还应当包括哪些内容？

2.1.2 患者问卷

国家中医药管理局
失眠针灸临床实践指南意见征询稿
（患者问卷）

省/直辖市/自治区_____   病程_____（年/月）

尊敬的各位患者，感谢您在百忙之中填写这份问卷。

为了协助国家中医药管理局标准化研究项目《失眠针灸临床实践指南》的顺利进行，使得这份指南具有最大程度上的实用性和针对性，现需要就相关针灸临床问题向您征询意见，请您逐项独立填写本问卷。对于您对本项目的支持，我们再次表示衷心的感谢。

填写说明：

1. 本问卷的征询对象为失眠患者。

2. 请根据您的真实感受独立填写本问卷。

3. 本问卷第一部分，只需在您觉得适当的表格内画√即可。例如，您"关注"失眠的"日常护理要点"，则只需在第6行对应"关注"的表格内画√。

4. 本问卷第二部分为开放性问题，请您将答案写在题目下面的空白处，如果空白不够，可另附页。

5. 填写本问卷时请您保证字迹清楚，容易辨认。

失眠针灸临床指南课题组
2010 年

第一部分

项目	不关注 0分	一般关注 1分	关注 2分	比较关注 3分	非常关注 4分
1. 症状					
2. 临床流行病（包括发病率、遗传性等）					
3. 易发人群					
4. 发病因素和机理					
5. 常见危险因素或诱发因素					
6. 日常护理要点					
7. 发病时的简单处理方法					
8. 针灸治疗的方法					
9. 针灸治疗的频率					
10. 针灸治疗的疗程					
11. 针灸治疗效果 对入睡困难的疗效					
对易醒或觉醒次数多的疗效					
对睡眠质量差的疗效					
对睡眠时间短的疗效					
对头昏、乏力、嗜睡、精神不振等伴随症状的疗效					
12. 病程长短与疗效之间的关系					
13. 针灸治疗的耐受性					
14. 针灸治疗的最佳时机					
15. 针灸治疗的复发性					
16. 针灸治疗的安全性					
17. 针灸治疗的不良反应					
18. 针灸治疗的禁忌证					
19. 针灸治疗期间的注意事项					
20. 针灸治疗的卫生经济学					
21. 其他配合治疗方法					

第二部分

1. 除了上述问题，您认为该指南中还应当包括哪些内容？

2. 您对于该问卷的改进和完善有何建议？

2.2 征询结果

1. 意见征询的范围涵盖了超过8个省市、自治区、直辖市，具体如下：

(1) 北京市：36 (37.9%)

(2) 江西省：5 (5.3%)

(3) 江苏省：5 (5.3%)

(4) 上海市：10 (10.5%)

(5) 广东省：7 (7.4%)

(6) 山东省：10 (10.5%)

(7) 浙江省：10 (10.5%)

(8) 四川省：8 (8.4%)

(9) 其他：4 (4.2%)

说明本问卷基本能够反映全国意见的状况。

2. 意见征询对象的职称情况分析如下：

(1) 主任医师/高级：18 (18.9%)

(2) 副主任医师/副高：26 (27.4%)

(3) 主治医师/中级：24 (25.3%)

(4) 住院医师/初级：27 (28.4%)

其中，高级职称所占比例达到46.3%，且中、初级职称人员所占比例比较均衡，体现了本问卷既多层次兼顾，又重点突出的调查原则。

3. 广大医生认为，在失眠的所有类型中，针灸治疗产生的疗效最可靠的三种类型分别是：

(1) 单纯性失眠：78 (82.1%)

(2) 更年期失眠：47 (49.5%)

(3) 精神疾病失眠：19 (20.0%)

4. 广大医生认为，失眠中最常见的五种证型分别是：

(1) 心脾两虚型：49 (51.6%)

(2) 心肾不交型：21 (22.1%)

(3) 肝郁化火型：21 (22.1%)

(4) 胃腑失和型：17 (17.9%)

（5）胆郁痰扰型：20（21.1%）

此外，也有医生认为，该病与跷脉（1.1%）失调关系密切。

5. 根据各位医生的经验，他们治疗失眠时，最常使用的穴位类型分别为：

（1）与"神"有关的穴：78（82.1%）

（2）背俞穴：38（40.0%）

（3）八脉交会穴：22（23.2%）

（4）辨证脏腑配穴：27（28.4%）

（5）手足部特定穴位：14（14.7%）

此外，也有医生认为，治疗该病时应当使用耳穴（1.1%）、跷脉穴（2.2%）以及灵龟八法（1.1%）。

6. 各位医生在治疗失眠时最常用的治疗手段分别是：

（1）针刺：93（97.9%）

（2）艾灸：29（30.5%）

（3）耳压：28（29.5%）

（4）拔罐：11（11.6%）

（5）其他：包括药物（3.3%）、灵龟八法（2.1%）和心理疏导（1.1%）。

7. 针对每一种类型的失眠，最佳的治疗方法分别是：

（1）单纯性失眠：针刺77（81.1%）、艾灸24（25.3%）、耳穴压丸29（30.5%）

（2）遗传性失眠：针刺37（38.9%）、艾灸11（11.6%）、耳穴压丸16（16.8%）

（3）更年期失眠：针刺64（67.4%）、艾灸22（23.2%）、耳穴压丸22（23.2%）

（4）产后失眠：针刺51（53.7%）、艾灸23（24.2%）、耳穴压丸20（21.1%）

（5）脑血管病失眠：针刺53（55.8%）、艾灸16（16.8%）、耳穴压丸21（22.1%）

（6）内科疾病失眠：针刺56（58.9%）、艾灸19（20.0%）、耳穴压丸22（23.2%）

（7）精神疾病失眠：针刺42（44.2%）、电针13（13.7%）、耳穴压丸12（12.6%）

（8）药物依赖性失眠：针刺36（37.9%）、电针14（14.7%）、耳穴压丸9（9.5%）

8. 有89.5%（85）的医生认为，针刺治疗失眠的同时应当配合使用其他疗法，最常用的疗法包括：

（1）中药：52（54.7%）

（2）足浴/足底按摩：26（27.4%）

（3）按摩推拿：14（14.7%）

（4）功能性仪器：14（14.7%）

（5）西药：17（17.9%）

9. 有80%（76）的医生认为，补泻在针灸治疗失眠中是重要的，最常用的补泻方法包括：

（1）泻阳补阴法：28（29.5%）

（2）平补平泻法：11（11.6%）

（3）补法：3（3.2%）

另外，一部分医生认为应当通过辨证决定补泻方法（11.6%）。

10. 有 53.7%（51）的医生认为，针灸治疗失眠最佳的治疗时间是 30 分钟。

11. 有 71.6%（68）的医生认为，针灸治疗失眠最佳的治疗频率是 1 天 1 次。

12. 有 56.8%（54）的医生认为，针灸治疗失眠的疗程应当是 10 次 1 个疗程。

13. 广大医生对本指南内容的关注程度如下：
（1）针灸选穴：322
（2）针灸方法及具体操作：301
（3）辨证分型：289
（4）针灸治疗原则：287
（5）临床表现：281
（6）中医诊断：281
（7）疗效及预后：273
（8）针灸介入时机：252
（9）疗效评价方法：248
（10）疗程及治疗频率：246
（11）西医诊断：244
（12）配合使用的其他中医方法：241
（13）危险因素/诱发因素：239
（14）注意事项：236
（15）禁忌证：234
（16）不良反应：227
（17）西医分型：217
（18）推荐方案的支持证据及其级别：211
（19）定义：188
（20）卫生经济学评价：179
（21）临床流行病情况：177

此外，对于该问卷，还有医生提出其他的建议，具体如下：①针灸治疗的疗效与疗程之间的关系问题。②关于心理暗示、诱导、催眠等影响因素。

3 疗效评价指标的分级

7~9 级	匹兹堡睡眠质量指数（PSQI）
	睡眠率（分值）
	阿森斯睡眠量表（AIS）（分值）
4~6 级	睡眠状况自评量表
	Epworth 评分
	失眠患者症状积分
	起效时间及疗程
	复发率
	无效率（《中医病证诊断疗效标准》）
1~3 级	其他指标

4 检索范围、检索策略及结果

4.1 检索范围

4.1.1 中文数据库

名称	网址
中文生物医学期刊文献数据库	http：//sinomed. cintcm. ac. cn/index. jsp
中国中医药信息网	http：//www. cintcm. com
中国知识资源总库（CNKI）	http：//www. cnki. net/
中国医院数字图书馆	http：//cnki. cintcm. ac. cn/kns50/chkd_ index. aspx
中国期刊全文数据库（世纪期刊）	http：//cnkigk. cintcm. ac. cn/kns50/
万方数据知识服务平台	http：//wanfang. cintcm. ac. cn：8088/
维普科技期刊全文数据库	http：//omcq4. gicp. net：90/index. asp
国家科技文献中心	http：//www. nstl. gov. cn/index. html
读秀学术搜索	http：//edu. duxiu. com/
谷歌学术搜索	http：//scholar. google. com. hk/schhp？hl＝zh－CN
《全国报刊索引》数据库－中医药专题（1949 年以前）	http：//192. 168. 200. 80：8090/

4.1.2 外文数据库

名称	网址/地址
PubMed	http：//pubmed. gov
EMBASE	医科院图书馆
西文生物医学期刊文献服务系统（FMJS）	http：//192. 168. 200. 35：8080/fmjs/index. jsp
国家科技文献中心	http：//www. nstl. gov. cn/index. html
循证医学全文数据库（EBMR）	http：//ovidsp. ovid. com/autologin. html
EBSCO 中西医结合全文数据库－ALT HEALTH WATCH	http：//search. ebscohost. com/

名称	网址/地址
OCLC《美国联机图书馆系统》	http：//firstsearch. oclc. org/
Socolar 开放存取资源一站式检索平台	http：//www. socolar. com/
National Guideline Clearinghouse 美国国家临床指南发布中心	http：//www. guideline. gov/

4.2 检索策略

4.2.1 中文现代文献

4.2.1.1 关键词

"失眠" OR "入睡和睡眠障碍" OR "睡眠障碍" OR "不寐" OR "少眠"。

"病因学" OR "影响因素" OR "发病原因" OR "诱因"。

"针灸" OR "针刺" OR "毫针" OR "灸" OR "电针" OR "耳针" OR "耳穴压丸" OR "水针" OR "皮肤针" OR "皮内针" OR "梅花针" OR "头针" OR "手足针" OR "腕踝针" OR "面针" OR "眼针" OR "温针" OR "刺血疗法" OR "放血疗法" OR "三棱针疗法" OR "蜂针" OR "火针疗法" OR "激光针刺" OR "激光穴位照射" OR "舌针" OR "穴位疗法" OR "穴位按压" OR "点穴" OR "敷脐" OR "拔罐" OR "走罐" OR "闪罐" OR "针药并用"。

"选穴" OR "取穴" OR "配穴" OR "处方，针灸" OR "针灸处方"。

"时间因素" OR "时间治疗学" OR "时间医学" OR "择时" OR "子午流注"。

4.2.1.2 检索式

（"失眠" OR "入睡和睡眠障碍" OR "睡眠障碍" OR "不寐" OR "少眠"）AND（"病因学" OR "影响因素" OR "发病原因" OR "诱因"）。

（"失眠" OR "入睡和睡眠障碍" OR "睡眠障碍" OR "不寐" OR "少眠"）AND（"针灸" OR "针刺" OR "毫针" OR "灸" OR "电针" OR "耳针" OR "耳穴" OR "水针" OR "穴位注射" OR "皮肤针" OR "皮内针" OR "梅花针" OR "头针" OR "手足针" OR "腕踝针" OR "面针" OR "眼针" OR "温针" OR "刺血" OR "放血" OR "三棱针" OR "蜂针" OR "火针" O "激光针刺" OR "激光穴位照射" OR "舌针" OR "穴位疗法" OR "敷脐" OR "拔罐" OR "走罐" OR "闪罐" OR "针药并用" OR "针药结合"）。

（"失眠" OR "入睡和睡眠障碍" OR "睡眠障碍" OR "不寐" OR "少眠"）AND（"选穴" OR "取穴" OR "配穴" OR "处方，针灸" OR "针灸处方"）。

（"失眠" OR "入睡和睡眠障碍" OR "睡眠障碍" OR "不寐" OR "少眠"）AND（"针灸" OR "针刺" OR "毫针" OR "灸" OR "电针" OR "耳针" OR "耳穴压丸" OR "水针" OR "皮肤针" OR "皮内针" OR "梅花针" OR "头针" OR "手足针" OR "腕踝针" OR "面针" OR "眼针" OR "温针" OR "刺血疗法" OR "放血疗法" OR "三棱针疗法" OR "蜂针" OR "火针疗法" OR "激光针刺" OR "激光穴位照射" OR "舌针" OR "穴位疗法" OR "穴位按压" OR "点" OR "敷脐" OR "拔罐" OR "走罐" OR "闪罐" OR "针药并用"）AND（"时间因素" OR "时间治疗学" OR "时间医学" OR "择时" OR "子午流注"）。

4.2.2 中文古代文献

"不寐" OR "不得眠" OR "不得卧" OR "不能眠" OR "失眠" OR "目不瞑" OR "无眠" OR "不眠" OR "少睡" OR "少寐" OR "不睡"。

4.2.3 英文文献

4.2.3.1 关键词

"Sleep Initiation and Maintenance Disorders" OR "Insomnia" OR "Sleeplessness" OR "Sleep Initiation Dysfunction".

"Etiology" OR "Causes" OR "Causality" OR "Epidemiologic Factors".

"Acupuncture" OR "Needling" OR "Moxibustion" OR "Electro – acupuncture" OR "Auricular Therapy" OR "Hydro – acupuncture" OR "Plum – blossom Needle therapy" OR "Intra – dermal Needle Therapy" OR "Needle Warming Therapy" OR "Bloodletting Therapy" OR "Three – edged Needle Therapy" OR "Bee – needles" OR "Fire – needle Therapy" OR "Laser" OR "Acupoint Therapy" OR "Acupressure" OR "Acupoint Sticking Therapy" OR "Auricular Point Sticking" OR "Cupping".

"Point Selection" OR "Acupoint Selection" OR "Point Combination" OR "Acupoint Combination" OR "Acupuncture – moxibustion Prescription" OR "Acupuncture Prescription" OR "Prescription Acupuncture – moxibustion".

"Time" OR "Time Factor" OR "Chronotherapeuties" OR "Chronomedicine" OR "Zi Wu Liu Zhu" OR "Ziwuliuzhu".

4.2.3.2 检索式

("Sleep Initiation and Maintenance Disorders" OR "Insomnia" OR "Sleeplessness" OR "Sleep Initiation Dysfunction") AND ("Etiology" OR "Causes" OR "Causality" OR "Epidemiologic Factors").

("Sleep Initiation and Maintenance Disorders" OR "Insomnia" OR "Sleeplessness" OR "Sleep Initiation Dysfunction") AND ("Acupuncture" OR "Needling" OR "Moxibustion" OR "Electro – acupuncture" OR "Auricular Therapy" OR "Hydro – acupuncture" OR "Plum – blossom Needle therapy" OR "Intra – dermal Needle Therapy" OR "Needle Warming Therapy" OR "Bloodletting Therapy" OR "Three – edged Needle Therapy" OR "Bee – needles" OR "Fire – needle Therapy" OR "Laser" OR "Acupoint Therapy" OR "Acupressure" OR "Acupoint Sticking Therapy" OR "Auricular Point Sticking" OR "Cupping").

("Sleep Initiation and Maintenance Disorders" OR "Insomnia" OR "Sleeplessness" OR "Sleep Initiation Dysfunction") AND ("Point Selection" OR "Acupoint Selection" OR "Point Combination" OR "Acupoint Combination" OR "Acupuncture – moxibustion Prescription" OR "Acupuncture Prescription" OR "Prescription Acupuncture – moxibustion").

("Sleep Initiation and Maintenance Disorders" OR "Insomnia" OR "Sleeplessness" OR "Sleep Initiation Dysfunction") AND ("Acupuncture" OR "Needling" OR "Moxibustion" OR "Electro – acupuncture" OR "Auricular Therapy" OR "Hydro – acupuncture" OR "Plum – blossom Needle therapy" OR "Intra – dermal Needle Therapy" OR "Needle Warming Therapy" OR "Bloodletting Therapy" OR "Three – edged Needle Therapy" OR "Bee – needles" OR "Fire – needle Therapy" OR "Laser" OR "Acupoint Therapy" OR "Acupressure" OR "Acupoint Sticking Therapy" OR "Auricular Point Sticking" OR "Cupping") AND ("Time" OR "Time Factor" OR "Chronotherapeuties" OR "Chronomedicine" OR "Zi Wu Liu Zhu" OR "Ziwuliuzhu").

4.3 检索结果

4.3.1 中文现代文献

中文现代文献检索结果

文献类型	随机对照试验	非随机同期对照试验	病例序列研究	个案报道	灰色文献
篇 数	214	114	408	39	0
共 计	775				

中文 RCT 文献风险评估结果

文献类型	真 RCT	假 RCT	拒绝回答	因故未回答	查无此人	邮箱未联系到	论文未联系到	无人应答	没有联系方式
数量	8	14	7	13	13	34	29	37	59
共计	214								

注：中文现代文献数量繁多，这里仅列出检索情况，后续外文文献、现代著作、古代文献编号与中文现代文献是接续关系。

4.3.2 外文现代文献

776 Edzard Ernst, Myeong Soo Lee & Tae－Young Choi. Acupuncture for insomnia An overview of systematic reviews. European Journal of General Practice, 2011, Early Online：1－8.

777 Jerome Sarris, GerardJ, Byrne. A systematic review of insomnia and complementary medicine. Sleep MedicineReviews, 2010, April：1－8.

778 Huijuan Cao, Xingfang Pan, Hua Li and Jianping Liu. Acupuncture for treatment of insomnia a systematic review of randomized controlled trials. The Journal of Alternative and Complementary Medicine. 2009, 15（11）：1171－1186.

779 Wing－Fai Yeung, Ka－Fai Chung, Yau－Kwong Leung, Shi－Ping Zhang, Andrew C. K. Law. Traditional needle acupuncture treatment for insomnia a systematic review of randomized controlled trials. Sleep Medicine, 2009（10）：694－704.

780 Wei Huang, Nancy Kutne, Donald L, Bliwise. A systematic review of the effects of acupuncture in treating insomnia. Sleep Medicine Reviews, 2009,（13）：73－104.

781 Agatha P Colbert, James Cleaver, Kimberly Ann Brown, etal. Magnets applied to acupuncture points as therapy － a literature review. Acupuncture in Medicine, 2008, 26（3）：160－170.

782 M. S. Lee, B. C. Shin, L. K. P. Suen, T. Y. Park, E. Ernst. Auricular acupuncture for insomnia a systematic review. International Journal of Clinical Practice, 2008, 62（11）：1744－1752.

783 Hai Yong Chen, Yan Shi, Chi Sun Ng, etal. Auricular acupuncture treatment for insomnia a systematic review. The Journal of Alternative and Complementary Medicine, 2007, 13（6）：669－676.

784 Cheuk DKL, Yeung J, Chung KF, Wong V. Acupuncture for insomnia. The Cochrane Collaboration. 2009.

785 Ramprasad Kalavapalli, Ravi Singareddy. Role of acupuncture in the treatment of insomnia a comprehensive review. Complementary Therapies in Clinical Practice, 2007,（13）：184－193.

786 Sohyune R. Sok, Judith A. Erlen, Kwuy Bun Kim. Effects of acupuncture therapy on insomnia. Journal of Advanced Nursing, 2003, 44（4）：375－384.

787 Felise S. Zollman, Eric B. Larson, Laura K. Wasek－Throm, etal. Acupuncture for Treatment of Insomnia in Patients With Traumatic Brain Injury A Pilot Intervention Study. Journal of Head Trauma Rehabilitation, 2011.

788 Wei Huang, Nancy Kutner, Donald L. Bliwise. Autonomic activation in insomnia the case for acupuncture. Journal of Clinical Sleep Medicine. 2011, 7 (11): 95 - 102.

789 Yen - Ying Kung, Cheryl C. H. Yang, Jen - Hwey Chiu, etal. The relationship of subjective sleep quality and cardiac autonomic nervous system in postmenopausal women with insomnia under auricular acupressure. The Journal of The North American Menopause Society, 2011, 18 (6): 1 - 8.

790 Gao Xi - yan, Ren Shan, Wang Pei - yu. Acupuncture treatment of insomnia by regulating the defensive - qi and strengthening the brain and the spinal cord. Journal of Traditional Chinese Medicine, 2010, 30 (3): 222 - 227.

791 Zhang Yue - feng, Ren Gui - fang & Zhang Xiu - chun. Acupuncture plus Cupping for Treating Insomnia in College Students. Journal of Traditional Chinese Medicine, 2010, 30 (3): 185 - 189.

792 Li Ling - feng & Lu Jian - hua. Clinical observation on acupuncture treatment of intractable insomnia. Journal of Traditional Chinese Medicine, 2010, 30 (1): 21 - 22.

793 Felise S. Zollman, Cherina Cyborski & Sylvia A. Duraski. Actigraphy for assessment of sleep in traumatic brain injury case series, review of the literature and proposed criteria for use. Brain Injury, 2010, 24 (5): 748 - 754.

794 Jia - Ling Sun, Mei - Sheng Sung, Mei - Yu Huang, etal. Effectiveness of acupressure for residents of long - term care facilities with insomnia a randomized controlled trial. International Journal of Nursing Studies, 2010, (47): 798 - 805.

795 Ciara M Hughes, Carey A McCullough, Ian Bradbury, etal. Acupuncture and reflexology for insomnia. Acupunct Med, 2009, 27: 163 - 168.

796 Seung Yeop Lee, Yong Hyeon Baek, Seong Uk Park, etal. Intradermal acupuncture on shen - men and nei - kuan acupoints improves insomnia in stroke patients by reducing the sympathetic nervous activity a randomized clinical trial. The American Journal of Chinese Medicine, 2009, 37 (6): 1013 - 1021.

797 Ying Chang, Miaoli, Yia - Ping Liu, etal. The effect on serotonin and MDA levels in depressed patients with insomnia when far - infrared rays are applied to acupoints. The American Journal of Chinese Medicine, 2009, 37 (5): 837 - 842.

798 Yeung WF. Electroacupuncture for Primary Insomnia A Randomized Controlled Trial. Sleep, 2009, 32 (8): 1039 - 1047.

799 Ju Yan - li, Chi Xu &Liu Jian - xin. Forty cases of insomnia treated by suspended moxibustion at Baihui (GV 20). Journal of Traditional Chinese Medicine, 2009, 29 (2): 95 - 96.

800 Huang Li - sha, Wang Dan - lin, Wang Cheng - wei, etal. The needle - rolling therapy for treatment of non - organic chronic insomnia in 90 cases. Journal of Traditional Chinese Medicine, 2009, 29 (1): 19 - 23.

801 Ling Li, Jiang Xin - mei, Xue Jin - wei, etal. Clinical study on the visceral differentiation - based acupuncture therapy for insomnia. Journal of Traditional Chinese Medicine, 2008, 28 (4): 270 - 273.

802 Huang Yong, Liao Xiao - ming, Li Xiao - xi, etal. Clinical observation on the effects of Bo's abdominal acupuncture in 40 cases of chronic fatigue syndrome. Journal of Traditional Chinese Medicine, 2008, 28 (4): 264 - 266.

803 Yao Y. Shieh, Fong Y. Tsai. Static magnetotherapy for the treatment of insomnia. Int. J. Electronic Healthcare, 2008, 4: 339 - 349.

804 R. Cerrone, L. Giani, B. Galbiati, etal. Efficacy of HT 7 point acupressure stimulation in the treatment of insomnia in cancer patients and in patients suffering from disorders other than cancer. Minerva Medica, 2008, 99 (6): 535 - 537.

805 Wang Xiao - yun, Yuan Song - hua, Yang Hong - yan, etal. Abdominal acupuncture for insomnia in women. Acupuncture amd Electro - Therapeutics Res. Int. J, 2008, 33: 33 - 41.

806 Mats Sjoling, Marianne Rolleri, Erling Englund. Auricular acupuncture versus sham acupuncture. The Journal of Alternarive and Complementary Medicine. 2008, 14 (1): 39 - 46.

807 Lv Ming, Liu Xiaoyan. Insomnia due to deficiency of both the heart and spleen treated by acupuncture – moxibustion and Chinese tuina. Journal of Traditional Chinese Medicine, 2008, 28 (1): 10 – 12.

808 Myeong Soo Lee. More about auricular acupuncture for insomnia.

809 Thomas Lundeberg, Iréne Lund. Did The Princess on the Pea′suffer from fibromyalgia syndrome. Acupuncture in Medicine, 2007, 25 (4): 184 – 197.

810 Nalaka S. Gooneratne. Complementary and alternative medicine for sleep disturbances in older adults. Clin Geriatr Med, 2008, 24: 121 – 138.

811 Kwuy Bun Kim, Sohyune R. Sok. Auricular acupuncture for insomnia. Journal of Gerontological Nursing, 2007, 23 – 28.

812 Liu Weizhe. Forty cases of insomnia treated by multi – output. Journal of Traditional Chinese Medicine, 2007, 27 (2): 106 – 107.

813 Luca Cabrini, Luigi Gioia, Marco Gemma, etal. Bispectral index evaluation of the sedative effect of acupuncture in healthy volunteers. Journal of Clinical Monitoring and Computing, 2006, 20: 311 – 315.

814 João Bosco Guerreiro da Silva, Mary Uchiyama Nakamura, José Antonio Cordeiro, et al. Acupuncture for insomnia in pregnancy. Acupuncture in Medicine, 2005, 23 (2): 47 – 51.

815 Young Suk Kim, Sang Ho Lee, Woo Sang Jung, etal. Intradermal acupuncture on shen – men and nei – kuan acupoints. The American Journal of Chinese Medicine, 2004, 32 (5): 771 – 778.

816 Shen Pei – wen. Two hundred cases of insomnia treated by otopoint pressure plus acupuncture. Journal of Traditional Chinese Medicine, 2004, 24 (3): 168 – 169.

817 Laura L. Murra, Hye – YoungKim. A review of select alternative treatment approaches for acquired neurogenic disorders relaxation therapy and acupuncture. Seminars in Speech and Language, 2004, 25 (2): 133 – 149.

818 D. Warren Spence, Leonid Kayumov, Adam Chen, etal. Acupuncture increases nocturnal melatonin secretion and reduces insomnia and anxiety. J Neuropsychiatry Clin Neurosci, 2004, 16 (1): 19 – 28.

819 Shi Dong – li. Acupuncture treatment of insomnia – – a report of 28 cases. Journal of Traditional Chinese Medicine, 2003, 23 (2): 136 – 137.

820 Zhang Qiu – ju. Clinical observation on acupuncture treatment of insomnia in 35 cases. Journal of Traditional Chinese Medicine, 2003, 23 (2): 125 – 126.

821 L. K. P. Suen, T. K. S. Wong, A. W. N. Leung, etal. The long – term effects of auricular therapy using magnetic pearls on elderly with insomnia. Complementary Therapies in Medicine, 2003, 11: 85 – 92.

822 Cui rui, Zhou De – an. Treatment of phlegm – and heat – induced insomnia by acupuncture in 120 cases. Journal of Traditional Chinese Medicine, 2003, 23 (1): 57 – 58.

823 Ravinder Mamtani, Andrea Cimino. A primer of complementary and alternative medicine and its relevance in the treatment of mental health problems. Psychiatric Quarterly, 2002, 73 (4): 367 – 381.

824 Dubravko Habek, Jasna Čerkez Habek, Ante Barbir. Using acupuncture to treat premenstrual syndrome. Arch Gynecol Obstet, 2002, 267: 23 – 26.

825 Lu Zeqiang. Scalp and body acupuncture for treatment of senile insomnia. Journal of Traditional Chinese Medicine, 2002, 22 (3): 193 – 194.

826 Michele M. Larzelere, Pamela Wiseman. Anxiety, depression, and insomnia. Prim Care Clin Office Pract, 2002, 29: 339 – 360.

827 Xin – qi Xu, Jamaica. Acupuncture in an outpatient clinic in China a comparison with the use of acupuncture in North A-merica. Southern Medical Journal, 2001, 94 (8): 813 – 816.

828 Yao Shuying. 46 cases of insomnia treated by semiconductor laser irradiation on auricular points. Journal of Traditional Chinese Medicine, 1999, 19 (4): 298 – 299.

829 Michael Woodward. Insomnia in the elderly. Australian Family Physician, 1999, 28 (7): 653 – 658.

830 Yinli Lin. Acupuncture treatment for insomnia and acupuncture analgesia. Psychiatry and Clinical Neurosciences, 1995, 49: 119 – 120.

831 Lian Nan, Yan Qingming. Insomnia treated by auricular pressing therapy. Journal of Traditional Chinese Medicine, 1990, 10 (3): 174 – 175.

832 Yang Cangliang. Clinical observation of 62 cases of insomnia treated by auricular point imbedding therapy. Journal of Tra-tional Chinese Medicine. 1988, 8 (3): 190 – 192.

833 Zhao Changxin. Lectures on formulating acupuncture prescriptions – selection and matching of acupoints. Acupuncture treatment of insomnia. Journal of Traditional Chinese Medicine, 1987, 7 (2): 151 – 152.

834 Ren Yi. 86 cases of insomnia treated by double point needling – daling through to waiguan. Journal of Traditional Chinese Medicine, 1985, 5 (1): 22.

4.3.3 现代著作

编号	作者	书名	页码	篇名	出版社	出版时间
835	贺普仁	《针灸三通法临床应用》	60～64	失眠（不寐）	北京科学技术文献出版社	1999
836	贺普仁	《毫针疗法图解》	48～49	不寐	山东科学技术出版社	1998
837	鲁之俊	《新编针灸学》	14～70	针灸刺激点的部位与作用	西南卫生书报出版社	1951
838	程莘农	《中国针灸学》	513～516	失眠（附：健忘）	人民卫生出版社	1964
839	陈湘生、张俊英	《金针王乐亭经验集》	157～159	论失眠健忘惊悸怔忡症	人民卫生出版社	2004
840	田从豁	《田从豁临床经验》	64～70	失眠	华文出版社	2000
841	田从豁	《针灸医学验集·田从豁》	555～561	失眠症	科学技术文献出版社	1985
842	田从豁、臧俊岐	《中国灸法集粹》	294～296	失眠症	辽宁科学技术出版社	1987
843	邱茂良	《针灸学》	226～227	不寐	上海科学技术出版社	1985
844	石学敏	《针灸治疗学》	186～191	不寐	人民卫生出版社	2001
845	石学敏	《中医针灸临床手册》	175		上海科学技术出版社	2004
846	石学敏	《当代针灸治疗学》	125～128	不寐	南开大学出版社	1998
847	承淡安	《承淡安针灸师承录》	137	痞寐门	人民军医出版社	2008
848	王宏才、郑真真	《针灸名家医案解读》	31～33	不寐	人民军医出版社	2008
849	石学敏	《石学敏针灸全集》	829～833	不寐（神经衰弱）	科学出版社	2006
850	承淡安、承为奋	《针灸真髓》	72		学苑出版社	2008
851	石学敏	《常见病实用针灸配方》	175～177	不寐（神经衰弱）	人民卫生出版社	2003
852	石学敏	《针灸推拿学》	265～267	不寐	中国中医药出版社	2002
853	陆瘦燕	《陆瘦燕针灸论著医案选》	215～216	失眠	人民卫生出版社	1984
854	刘志顺	《田从豁》	97～100	失眠	中国中医药出版社	2009
855	承淡安	《中国针灸学》	100～101	失眠	人民卫生出版社	1955
856	承淡安	《中国针灸治疗学》	370～374	神经衰弱	中国针灸学研究社	1937

4.3.4 古代文献

编号	书名	作者	版本	编码
857	《针灸集成》	清·廖润鸿	清光绪五年己卯 1879 京门琉璃厂宝名斋刻本	寅 11/1874/1/1
858	《针灸大成》	明·杨继洲	清嘉庆六年辛酉 1801 经纶堂重刻本	寅 11/1601/1/1
859	《勉学堂针灸集成》	清·廖润鸿	清光绪五年己卯 1879 京门琉璃厂宝名斋刻本	寅 11/1874/1/1
860	《神灸经纶》	清·吴亦鼎	中医古籍出版社 1983 版	7 – 80013 – 109 – 2/R. 109
861	《针灸甲乙经》	晋·皇甫谧	清光绪十二年乙酉 1885 存存轩刻本	寅 11/0282/1/1
862	《普济方》	明·朱木肃	据文朔阁四库全书本抄	巳 3/1406/2/22
863	《针灸聚英》	明·高武	明嘉靖十六年丁酉 1537 陶师文刻本	寅 11/1529/2/21
864	《刺灸心法要诀》	清·吴谦	清翻刻医宗金鉴丛书本	亥 22/1742/1/1
865	《类经图翼》	明·张介宾	明天启四年甲子 1624 天德堂刻本	丑 41/1622/1/1
866	《针灸资生经》	宋·王执中	见影抄文朔阁四库全书医家类十二种	亥 11/1782/2/2
867	《西方子明堂灸经》	元·西方子	明正德十年乙亥 1515 山西平阳府刻本	寅 41/1368/1/1
868	《神应经》	明·陈会	957 年据日本正保二年乙酉 1645 刻本抄	寅 11/1435/1/1
869	《针灸逢源》	清·李学川	嘉庆二十二年丁丑 1817 刻本	寅 11/1817/1/1
870	《针方六集》	明·吴昆	中华医学名著宝库 1999 版	7 – 80114 – 292 – 6

5 文献质量评估结论

abdominal acupuncture combined with acupuncture for insomnia

Author（s）：

Date：2013 −03 −22

Question：Should abdominal acupuncture combined with acupuncture be used for insomnia?

Settings：

Bibliography：

No of studies	Quality assessment						No of patients		Effect			Quality	Importance
	Design	Risk of bias	Inconsistency	Indirectness	Imprecision	Other considerations	Abdominal acupuncture combined with acupuncture	Control	Relative (95% CI)	Absolute			
PSQI ineffect rate −774													
1	observational studies[1]	serious[1]	no serious inconsistency	no serious indirectness	serious	reporting bias[2]	15/80 (18.8%)	−	−	−	⊕○○○ VERY LOW	CRITICAL

1 case series.

2 a single study.

abdominal acupuncture combined with auricular needle for insomnia

Author (s) :

Date: 2013 – 03 – 22

Question: Should abdominal acupuncture combined with auricular needle be used for insomnia?

Settings:

Bibliography:

No of studies	Quality assessment						No of patients		Effect		Quality	Importance
	Design	Risk of bias	Inconsistency	Indirectness	Imprecision	Other considerations	Abdominal acupuncture combined with auricular needle	Control	Relative (95% CI)	Absolute		
sleep rate – 769, 770												
2	observational studies[1]	serious[1]	no serious inconsistency	no serious indirectness	very serious	reporting bias[2]	4/64 (6.3%)	-	-	-	⊕○○○ VERY LOW	CRITICAL
ineffect rate – 771												
1	observational studies[1]	serious[1]	no serious inconsistency	no serious indirectness	very serious	reporting bias[3]	2/52 (3.8%)	-	-	-	⊕○○○ VERY LOW	IMPORTANT
ineffect rate (other criteria) – 772, 773												
2	observational studies[1]	serious[4]	no serious inconsistency	no serious indirectness	very serious	reporting bias[5]	4/68 (5.9%)	-	-	-	⊕○○○ VERY LOW	NOT IMPORTANT

1 case series.

2 the number is small and the authors are same.

3 a single study.

4 RCTs failing to connect with authors.

5 the number of studies is small.

acupuncture combined with auricular acupuncture for insomnia

Author (s):
Date: 2013 – 03 – 22
Question: Should acupuncture combined with auricular acupuncture be used for insomnia?
Settings:
Bibliography:

| No of studies | Quality assessment | | | | | | No of patients | | Effect | | Quality | Importance |
	Design	Risk of bias	Inconsistency	Indirectness	Imprecision	Other considerations	Acupuncture combined with auricular acupuncture	Control	Relative (95% CI)	Absolute		
Epworth – 588 (range of scores: 0 – 21; Better indicated by lower values)												
1	observational studies[1]	serious[2]	no serious inconsistency	no serious indirectness	serious	reporting bias[3]	29	–	–	–	⊕○○○ VERY LOW	IMPORTANT
PSQI – 588 – 598 (range of scores: 0 – 21; Better indicated by lower values)												
11	observational studies[1]	serious[2]	no serious inconsistency	no serious indirectness	serious	reporting bias[4]	474	–	–	–	⊕○○○ VERY LOW	CRITICAL
sleep rate – 594, 595······613												
14	observational studies[1]	serious[1,2]	no serious inconsistency	no serious indirectness	very serious	none	64/932 (6.9%)	–	–	–	⊕○○○ VERY LOW	CRITICAL
ineffect rate – 589, 590······635 (follow – up 4 – 8 weeks)												
26	observational studies[1]	serious[1,2]	no serious inconsistency	no serious indirectness	very serious	none	128/2107 (6.1%)	–	–	–	⊕○○○ VERY LOW	IMPORTANT
ineffect rate (other criteria) – 591, 636 – 693 (follow – up 2 – 12 months)												
59	observational studies[1]	serious[1,2]	no serious inconsistency	no serious indirectness	very serious	none	186/3691 (5%)	–	–	–	⊕○○○ VERY LOW	NOT IMPORTANT

1 case series.
2 a RCT failing to connect with the author.
3 a single study.
4 the number of studies is small and some authors are same.

acupuncture combined with bleeding for insomnia

Author (s):
Date: 2013 –03 –22
Question: Should acupuncture combined with bleeding be used for insomnia?
Settings:
Bibliography:

No of studies	Quality assessment						No of patients		Effect		Quality	Importance
	Design	Risk of bias	Inconsistency	Indirectness	Imprecision	Other considerations	Acupuncture combined with bleeding	Control	Relative (95% CI)	Absolute		
AIS –752 (range of scores: 0 –48; Better indicated by lower values)												
1	observational studies[1]	serious[2]	no serious inconsistency	no serious indirectness	serious	reporting bias[3]	29	-	-	-	⊕○○○ VERY LOW	CRITICAL
PSQI –753 (range of scores: 0 –21; Better indicated by lower values)												
1	observational studies[1]	serious[2]	no serious inconsistency	no serious indirectness	serious	reporting bias[3]	63	-	-	-	⊕○○○ VERY LOW	CRITICAL
sleep rate –757												
1	observational studies[1]	serious[2]	no serious inconsistency	no serious indirectness	very serious	reporting bias[3]	3/32 (9.4%)	-	-	-	⊕○○○ VERY LOW	CRITICAL
ineffect rate –752, 753, 758												
3	observational studies[1]	serious[1,2]	no serious inconsistency	no serious indirectness	very serious	reporting bias[4]	5/100 (5%)	-	-	-	⊕○○○ VERY LOW	IMPORTANT
ineffect rate (other criteria) –759, 760 (follow –up mean 6 months)												
2	observational studies[1]	serious[1,2]	no serious inconsistency	no serious indirectness	very serious	reporting bias[4]	1/77 (1.3%)	-	-	-	⊕○○○ VERY LOW	NOT IMPORTANT

1 case series.
2 a RCT failing to connect with the author.
3 a single study.
4 the number of studies is small.

acupuncture combined with cupping for insomnia

Author (s):

Date: 2013 – 03 – 22

Question: Should acupuncture combined with cupping be used for insomnia?

Settings:

Bibliography:

		Quality assessment					No of patients		Effect			
No of studies	Design	Risk of bias	Inconsistency	Indirectness	Imprecision	Other considerations	Acupuncture combined with cupping	Control	Relative (95% CI)	Absolute	Quality	Importance
SRSS – 694, 695 (range of scores: 10 – 50; Better indicated by lower values)												
2	observational studies[1]	serious[2]	no serious inconsistency	no serious indirectness	serious	reporting bias[3]	104	-	-	-	⊕◯◯◯ VERY LOW	IMPORTANT
sleep rate – 696 – 699												
4	observational studies[1]	serious[1,2]	no serious inconsistency	no serious indirectness	serious	reporting bias[4]	6/194 (3.1%)	-	-	-	⊕◯◯◯ VERY LOW	CRITICAL
ineffect rate – 694, 695……704												
7	observational studies[1]	serious[1,2]	no serious inconsistency	no serious indirectness	serious	reporting bias[4]	26/297 (8.8%)	-	-	-	⊕◯◯◯ VERY LOW	IMPORTANT
ineffect rate (other criteria) – 705 – 716 (follow – up mean 6 months)												
12	observational studies[1]	serious[1,2]	no serious inconsistency	no serious indirectness	very serious	none	32/636 (5%)	-	-	-	⊕◯◯◯ VERY LOW	NOT IMPORTANT

1 case series.

2 RCTs failing to connect with authors.

3 the number of studies is small, and the authors are same.

4 the number of studies is small, and the author of 2 of them are same.

acupuncture combined with dermal needle for insomnia

Author (s) :

Date: 2013 – 03 – 22

Question: Should acupuncture combined with dermal needle be used for insomnia?

Settings :

Bibliography :

No of studies	Quality assessment						No of patients		Effect		Quality	Importance
	Design	Risk of bias	Inconsistency	Indirectness	Imprecision	Other considerations	Acupuncture combined with dermal needle	Control	Relative (95% CI)	Absolute		
ineffect rate (other criteria) – 761 – 763												
3	observational studies[1]	serious[1]	no serious inconsistency	no serious indirectness	very serious	reporting bias[2]	9/141 (6. 4%)	-	-	-	⊕○○○ VERY LOW	NOT IMPORTANT

1 case series.

2 the number of studies is small.

acupuncture combined with moxibustion for insomnia

Author (s):

Date: 2013 -03 -22

Question: Should acupuncture combined with moxibustion be used for insomnia?

Settings:

Bibliography:

No of studies	Quality assessment						No of patients		Effect		Quality	Importance
	Design	Risk of bias	Inconsistency	Indirectness	Imprecision	Other considerations	Acupuncture combined with moxibustion	Control	Relative (95% CI)	Absolute		
PSQI ineffect rate - 717, 718												
2	observational studies[1]	serious[1,2]	no serious inconsistency	no serious indirectness	serious	reporting bias[3]	6/42 (14.3%)	-	-	-	⊕○○○ VERY LOW	CRITICAL
SRSS - 719 (range of scores: 10 - 50; Better indicated by lower values)												
1	observational studies[1]	serious[2]	no serious inconsistency	no serious indirectness	very serious	reporting bias[4]	30	-	-	-	⊕○○○ VERY LOW	IMPORTANT
sleep rate - 723												
1	observational studies[1]	serious[2]	no serious inconsistency	no serious indirectness	very serious	reporting bias[4]	2/33 (6.1%)	-	-	-	⊕○○○ VERY LOW	CRITICAL
ineffect rate - 724 - 728												
5	observational studies[1]	serious[1,2]	no serious inconsistency	no serious indirectness	serious	reporting bias[5]	11/223 (4.9%)	-	-	-	⊕○○○ VERY LOW	IMPORTANT
ineffect rate (other criteria) - 729 - 736												
8	observational studies[1]	serious[1]	no serious inconsistency	no serious indirectness	very serious	none	68/552 (12.3%)	-	-	-	⊕○○○ VERY LOW	NOT IMPORTANT

1 case series.

2 a RCT failing to connect with author.

3 the authors are same.

4 a single study.

5 the number of studies is small.

acupuncture combined with point application for insomnia

Author (s) :

Date: 2013 – 03 – 22

Question: Should acupuncture combined with point application be used for insomnia?

Settings:

Bibliography:

No of studies	Quality assessment						No of patients		Effect		Quality	Importance
	Design	Risk of bias	Inconsistency	Indirectness	Imprecision	Other considerations	Acupuncture combined with point application	Control	Relative (95% CI)	Absolute		
ineffect – 764, 765 (follow – up mean 2 months)												
2	observational studies[1]	serious[2]	no serious inconsistency	no serious indirectness	very serious	reporting bias[3]	16/201 (8%)	-	-	-	⊕◯◯◯ VERY LOW	IMPORTANT
ineffect rate (other criteria) – 767, 768												
2	observational studies[1]	serious[1]	no serious inconsistency	no serious indirectness	very serious	reporting bias[3]	15/218 (6.9%)	-	-	-	⊕◯◯◯ VERY LOW	NOT IMPORTANT

1 case series.

2 a RCT failing to connect with the author.

3 the number of studies is small.

acupuncture combined with point injection for insomnia

Author（s）：

Date：2013 – 03 – 22

Question：Should acupuncture combined with point injection be used for insomnia?

Settings：

Bibliography：

| No of studies | Quality assessment | | | | | | No of patients | | Effect | | Quality | Importance |
	Design	Risk of bias	Inconsistency	Indirectness	Imprecision	Other considerations	Acupuncture combined with point injection	Control	Relative (95% CI)	Absolute		
PSQI – 737（follow – up 6 weeks；range of scores：0 – 21；Better indicated by lower values）												
1	observational studies[1]	serious[2]	no serious inconsistency	no serious indirectness	serious	reporting bias[3]	30	-	-	-	⊕◯◯◯ VERY LOW	CRITICAL
sleep rate – 738, 739												
2	observational studies[1]	serious[1,2]	no serious inconsistency	no serious indirectness	serious	reporting bias[4]	2/88 (2. 3%)	-	-	-	⊕◯◯◯ VERY LOW	CRITICAL
ineffect rate – 737, 740 – 745												
7	observational studies[1]	serious[1,2]	no serious inconsistency	no serious indirectness	very serious	reporting bias[4]	40/449 (8. 9%)	-	-	-	⊕◯◯◯ VERY LOW	IMPORTANT
ineffect rate（other criteria） – 746 – 751												
6	observational studies[1]	serious[1,2]	no serious inconsistency	no serious indirectness	very serious	reporting bias[4]	8/1063 (0. 75%)	-	-	-	⊕◯◯◯ VERY LOW	NOT IMPORTANT

1 case series.

2 a RCT failing to connect with author.

3 a single study.

4 the number of studies is small.

auricular for insomnia

Author (s):

Date: 2013 – 03 – 16

Question: Should auricular be used for insomnia?

Settings:

Bibliography:

No of studies	Quality assessment						No of patients		Effect		Quality	Importance
	Design	Risk of bias	Inconsistency	Indirectness	Imprecision	Other considerations	Auricular	Control	Relative (95% CI)	Absolute		
PSQI – 54, 67, 68, 91, 96 – 98, 103 (measured with: PSQI scale; range of scores: 0 – 21; Better indicated by lower values)												
8	observational studies[1]	serious[1]	no serious inconsistency	no serious indirectness	serious	none[2]	361	-	-	-	⊕○○○ VERY LOW	CRITICAL
ineffect rate – 39, 53, 54, 67……167												
15	observational studies[1]	serious[1]	no serious inconsistency	no serious indirectness	serious	strong associ-ation3	85/847 (10%)	-	-	-	⊕○○○ VERY LOW	IMPORTANT
sleep time – 50, 121, 125 (Better indicated by higher values)												
3	observational studies[1]	serious[1]	no serious inconsistency	no serious indirectness	very serious	reporting bias[4]	210	-	-	-	⊕○○○ VERY LOW	IMPORTANT
sleep rate – 40, 44, 61, 85, 140 (assessed with: sleep time/ time on bed)												
5	observational studies[1]	serious[1]	no serious inconsistency	no serious indirectness	serious	reporting bias[5]	343/378 (90.7%)	-	-	-	⊕○○○ VERY LOW	CRITICAL
AIS – 68 (range of scores: 0 – 48; Better indicated by lower values)												
1	observational studies[1]	serious[1,6]	no serious inconsistency	no serious indirectness	serious	reporting bias[7]	32	-	-	-	⊕○○○ VERY LOW	CRITICAL

SRSS – 151

No of studies	Design	Risk of bias	Inconsistency	Indirectness	Imprecision	Other considerations	Balance acupuncture	Control	Relative (95% CI)	Absolute	Quality	Importance
1	observational studies[1]	serious[6]	no serious inconsistency	no serious indirectness	serious	reporting bias[7]	26/30 (86. 7%)	–	–	–	⊕○○○ VERY LOW	IMPORTANT
ineffect rate (other criteria) – 35, 37, 37·····168 (follow – up mean 3. 5 months)
94	observational studies[1]	serious[1,6]	no serious inconsistency	no serious indirectness	serious	strong associ- ation[2]	417/6245 (6. 7%)	–	–	–	⊕○○○ VERY LOW	NOT IMPORTANT

1 case series.

2 the number of studies is large, and the authors are from different department.

3 the studies are similar, and the case numbers are large.

4 the authors of 2 of them are from the same hospital, and the content of the articles are similar.

5 the number of studies is small.

6 a RCT failing to connect the author.

7 a single study.

balance acupuncture for insomnia

Author (s):

Date: 2013 – 03 – 19

Question: Should balance acupuncture be used for insomnia?

Settings:

Bibliography:

	Quality assessment						No of patients		Effect		Quality	Importance
No of studies	Design	Risk of bias	Inconsistency	Indirectness	Imprecision	Other considerations	Balance acupuncture	Control	Relative (95% CI)	Absolute		
1	observational studies[1]	serious[1]	no serious inconsistency	no serious indirectness	very serious	reporting bias[2]	3/106 (2. 8%)	–	–	–	⊕○○○ VERY LOW	IMPORTANT
ineffect rate – 207

1 case series.

2 a single study.

bleeding be used for insomnia

Author（s）：

Date：2013 – 03 – 19

Question：Should bleeding be used for insomnia?

Settings：

Bibliography：

| No of studies | Quality assessment | | | | | | No of patients | | Effect | | Quality | Importance |
	Design	Risk of bias	Inconsistency	Indirectness	Imprecision	Other considerations	Bleeding	Control	Relative (95% CI)	Absolute		
PSQI – 192（range of scores：0 – 21；Better indicated by lower values）												
1	observational studies[1]	serious[2]	no serious inconsistency	no serious indirectness	no serious imprecision	reporting bias[3]	85	-	-	-	⊕○○○ VERY LOW	CRITICAL
ineffect rate – 192												
1	observational studies[1]	serious[2]	no serious inconsistency	no serious indirectness	serious	reporting bias[3]	3/85 (3.5%)	-	-	-	⊕○○○ VERY LOW	IMPORTANT
sleep rate – 193												
1	observational studies[1]	serious[2]	no serious inconsistency	no serious indirectness	serious	reporting bias[3]	1/24 (4.2%)	-	-	-	⊕○○○ VERY LOW	CRITICAL
ineffect rate（other criteria）– 190，191												
2	observational studies[1]	serious[1]	no serious inconsistency	no serious indirectness	serious	reporting bias[4]	22/308 (7.1%)	-	-	-	⊕○○○ VERY LOW	NOT IMPORTANT

1 case series.

2 a RCT failing to connect with the author.

3 a single study.

4 the number of study is small.

cupping and scraping therapy for insomnia

Author (s) :

Date: 2013 – 03 – 19

Question: Should cupping and scraping therapy be used for insomnia?

Settings:

Bibliography:

No of studies	Quality assessment						No of patients		Effect		Quality	Importance
	Design	Risk of bias	Inconsistency	Indirectness	Imprecision	Other considerations	Cupping and scraping therapy	Control	Relative (95% CI)	Absolute		
AIS – cupping – 215 (follow – up mean 2 weeks; range of scores: 0 – 48; Better indicated by lower values)												
1	observational studies[1]	serious[2]	no serious inconsistency	no serious indirectness	serious	reporting bias[3]	36	–	–	–	⊕○○○ VERY LOW	CRITICAL
SRSS – cupping – 216 (range of scores: 10 – 50; Better indicated by lower values)												
1	observational studies[1]	serious[2]	no serious inconsistency	no serious indirectness	serious	reporting bias[3]	52	–	–	–	⊕○○○ VERY LOW	IMPORTANT
ineffect rate – cupping – 216												
1	observational studies[1]	serious[2]	no serious inconsistency	no serious indirectness	very serious	reporting bias[3]	4/52 (7.7%)	–	–	–	⊕○○○ VERY LOW	IMPORTANT
ineffect rate (other criteria) – cupping – 219 – 222 (follow – up mean 1 months)												
4	observational studies[1]	serious[1]	no serious inconsistency	no serious indirectness	very serious	reporting bias[4]	11/197 (5.6%)	–	–	–	⊕○○○ VERY LOW	NOT IMPORTANT
sleep rate – scraping – 223, 224												
2	observational studies[1]	serious[1]	no serious inconsistency	no serious indirectness	very serious	reporting bias[5]	0/22 (0%)	–	–	–	⊕○○○ VERY LOW	CRITICAL

Continued

No of studies	Design	Risk of bias	Inconsistency	Indirectness	Imprecision	Other considerations		Effect rate	Control	Relative (95% CI)	Absolute	Quality	Importance
ineffect rate (other criteria) – scraping –226													
1	observational studies[1]	serious[2]	no serious inconsistency	no serious indirectness	very serious	reporting bias[3]		4/52 (7.7%)	-	-	-	⊕○○○ VERY LOW	NOT IMPORTANT

1 case series.
2 a RCT failing to connect with author.
3 a single study.
4 the number of studies is small.
5 the authors of these studies are the same.

dermal needle for insomnia

Author (s) :

Date: 2013 – 03 – 19

Question: Should dermal needle be used for insomnia?

Settings:

Bibliography:

No of studies	Quality assessment						No of patients		Effect		Quality	Importance
	Design	Risk of bias	Inconsistency	Indirectness	Imprecision	Other considerations	Dermal needle	Control	Relative (95% CI)	Absolute		
ineffect rate –199												
1	observational studies[1]	serious[1]	no serious inconsistency	no serious indirectness	very serious	reporting bias[2]	2/50 (4%)	-	-	-	⊕○○○ VERY LOW	IMPORTANT
ineffect rate (other criteria) –200 – 206 (follow – up 3 – 6 months)												
7	observational studies[1]	serious[1]	no serious inconsistency	no serious indirectness	very serious	reporting bias[3]	17/284 (6%)	-	-	-	⊕○○○ VERY LOW	NOT IMPORTANT

1 case series.
2 a single study.
3 the number of studies is small.

eye acupuncture for insomnia

Author（s）：

Date：2013 – 03 – 19

Question：Should eye acupuncture be used for insomnia ?

Settings：

Bibliography：

No of studies	Design	Risk of bias	Inconsistency	Indirectness	Imprecision	Other considerations	Eye acupuncture	Control	Relative (95% CI)	Absolute	Quality	Importance
PSQI – 208 (range of scores: 0 – 21; Better indicated by lower values)												
1	observational studies[1]	serious[2]	no serious inconsistency	no serious indirectness	serious	reporting bias[3]	30	–	–	–	⊕◯◯◯ VERY LOW	CRITICAL
ineffect rate – 208, 209												
2	observational studies[1]	serious[4]	no serious inconsistency	no serious indirectness	very serious	reporting bias[5]	6/70 (8.6%)	–	–	–	⊕◯◯◯ VERY LOW	IMPORTANT
ineffect rate (other criteria) – 210												
1	observational studies[1]	serious[2]	no serious inconsistency	no serious indirectness	very serious	reporting bias[3]	10/68 (14.7%)	–	–	–	⊕◯◯◯ VERY LOW	NOT IMPORTANT

1 case series.

2 a RCT failing to connect with the author.

3 a single study.

4 RCTS failing to connect with authors.

5 the number of studies is small.

interdermal needle for insomnia

Author (s) :

Date : 2013 – 03 – 20

Question : Should interdermal needle be used for insomnia?

Settings :

Bibliography :

No of studies	Quality assessment						No of patients		Effect		Quality	Importance
	Design	Risk of bias	Inconsistency	Indirectness	Imprecision	Other considerations	Interdermal needle	Control	Relative (95% CI)	Absolute		
ineffect rate (other criteria) – 232 – 235												
4	observational studies[1]	serious[2]	no serious inconsistency	no serious indirectness	very serious	reporting bias[3]	19/289 (6.6%)	-	-	-	⊕◯◯◯ VERY LOW	NOT IMPORTANT

1 case series.

2 case seires and RCT failing to connect with author.

3 the number of studies is small.

magnetic needle for insomnia

Author (s):

Date: 2013－03－19

Question: Should magnetic needle be used for insomnia?

Settings:

Bibliography:

Quality assessment							No of patients		Effect		Quality	Importance
No of studies	Design	Risk of bias	Inconsistency	Indirectness	Imprecision	Other considerations	Magnetic needle	Control	Relative (95% CI)	Absolute		
PSQI－227 (range of scores: 0－21; Better indicated by lower values)												
1	observational studies[1]	serious[2]	no serious inconsistency	no serious indirectness	serious	reporting bias[3]	68	-	-	-	⊕○○○ VERY LOW	CRITICAL
ineffect rate (other criteria) －228 (follow－up mean 1 months)												
1	observational studies[1]	serious[2]	no serious inconsistency	no serious indirectness	very serious	reporting bias[3]	0/30 (0%)	-	-	-	⊕○○○ VERY LOW	NOT IMPORTANT

1 case series.

2 a RCT failing to connect with the author.

3 a single study.

moxibustion for insomnia

Author (s) :

Date: 2013 – 03 – 19

Question: Should moxibustion be used for insomnia?

Settings :

Bibliography :

No of studies	Quality assessment						No of patients		Effect		Quality	Importance
	Design	Risk of bias	Inconsistency	Indirectness	Imprecision	Other considerations	Moxibustion	Control	Relative (95% CI)	Absolute		
PSQI ineffect rate – 169, 180												
2	observational studies[1]	serious[1]	no serious inconsistency	no serious indirectness	serious	reporting bias[2]	6/78 (7.7%)	-	-	-	⊕○○○ VERY LOW	CRITICAL
ineffect rate – 181, 189												
2	observational studies[1]	serious[3]	no serious inconsistency	no serious indirectness	serious	reporting bias[2]	6/85 (7.1%)	-	-	-	⊕○○○ VERY LOW	IMPORTANT
ineffect rate (other criteria) – 171, 173⋯⋯188 (follow – up 0 – 12 months)												
13	observational studies[1]	serious[1]	no serious inconsistency	no serious indirectness	serious	none	51/779 (6.5%)	-	-	-	⊕○○○ VERY LOW	NOT IMPORTANT
sleep rate – 187												
1	observational studies[1]	serious[1]	no serious inconsistency	no serious indirectness	serious	reporting bias[4]	36/40 (90%)	-	-	-	⊕○○○ VERY LOW	CRITICAL

1 case series.

2 the number of studies is small.

3 they are RCTS failing to connet with authors.

4 single study.

normal acupuncture for insomnia

Author (s):

Date: 2013 – 03 – 22

Question: Should normal acupuncture be used for insomnia?

Settings:

Bibliography:

No of studies	Quality assessment						No of patients		Effect		Quality	Importance
	Design	Risk of bias	Inconsistency	Indirectness	Imprecision	Other considerations	Normal acupuncture	Control	Relative (95% CI)	Absolute		
AIS – 276 – 279 (range of scores: 0 – 48; Better indicated by lower values)												
4	observational studies[1]	serious[2]	no serious inconsistency	no serious indirectness	no serious imprecision	reporting bias[3]	142	–	–	–	⊕◯◯◯ VERY LOW	CRITICAL
Epworth – 280 – 285 (follow – up 4 – 6 weeks; range of scores: 0 – 21; Better indicated by lower values)												
6	observational studies[1]	serious[2]	no serious inconsistency	no serious indirectness	no serious imprecision	reporting bias[3],[4]	187	–	–	–	⊕◯◯◯ VERY LOW	IMPORTANT
PSQI ineffect rate – 307, 327 – 330 (follow – up 1 – 6 months)												
5	observational studies[1]	serious[1],[2]	no serious inconsistency	no serious indirectness	very serious	reporting bias[3],[4]	38/287 (13.2%)	–	–	–	⊕◯◯◯ VERY LOW	CRITICAL
SCL – 90 – 310, 318 (range of scores: 0 – 360; Better indicated by lower values)												
2	observational studies[1]	serious[2]	no serious inconsistency	no serious indirectness	serious	reporting bias[5]	86	–	–	–	⊕◯◯◯ VERY LOW	NOT IMPORTANT
PSQI – 276, 278……326 (follow – up 4 – 24 weeks; range of scores: 0 – 21; Better indicated by lower values)												
48	observational studies[1]	serious[1],[2]	no serious inconsistency	no serious indirectness	no serious imprecision	strong association[6]	1655	–	–	–	⊕◯◯◯ LOW	CRITICAL

Continued

SDRS – 331, 332 (range of scores: 0 – 21; Better indicated by lower values)

3	observational studies[1]	serious[2]	no serious inconsistency	no serious indirectness	serious	reporting bias[3]	61	–	–	–	⊕◯◯◯ VERY LOW	NOT IMPORTANT

SPIEGEL – 333 (range of scores: 0 – 42; Better indicated by lower values)

1	observational studies[1]	serious[2]	no serious inconsistency	no serious indirectness	serious	reporting bias[7]	30	–	–	–	⊕◯◯◯ VERY LOW	NOT IMPORTANT

SF – 36 – 281 (follow – up mean 6 weeks; range of scores: 0 – 100; Better indicated by higher values)

1	observational studies[1]	serious[2]	no serious inconsistency	no serious indirectness	serious	reporting bias[7]	28	–	–	–	⊕◯◯◯ VERY LOW	NOT IMPORTANT

SQ – 334 – 335 (range of scores: 0 – 42; Better indicated by lower values)

2	observational studies[1]	serious[2]	no serious inconsistency	no serious indirectness	serious	reporting bias[3]	58	–	–	–	⊕◯◯◯ VERY LOW	NOT IMPORTANT

SRSS – 336 (range of scores: 10 – 50; Better indicated by lower values)

1	observational studies[1]	serious[2]	no serious inconsistency	no serious indirectness	serious	reporting bias[7]	87	–	–	–	⊕◯◯◯ VERY LOW	IMPORTANT

SSDS – 331 (range of scores: 0 – 30; Better indicated by lower values)

1	observational studies[1]	serious[2]	no serious inconsistency	no serious indirectness	serious	reporting bias[7]	31	–	–	–	⊕◯◯◯ VERY LOW	IMPORTANT

SSS – 281 (follow – up mean 6 weeks; Better indicated by lower values)

1	observational studies[1]	serious[2]	no serious inconsistency	no serious indirectness	serious	reporting bias[7]	28	–	–	–	⊕◯◯◯ VERY LOW	NOT IMPORTANT

awaking times –370 (follow – up 6 –36 months; Better indicated by lower values)

	observational studies[1]	serious[1]	no serious inconsistency	no serious indirectness	serious	reporting bias[7]	68	–	–	–	⊕◯◯◯ VERY LOW	NOT IMPORTANT
1												

clinical symotpms integrals –319 (range of scores: 0 –21; Better indicated by lower values)

	observational studies[1]	serious[2]	no serious inconsistency	no serious indirectness	serious	reporting bias[7]	30	–	–	–	⊕◯◯◯ VERY LOW	IMPORTANT
1												

sleep time –314, 315······409 (follow – up 6 –36 weeks; Better indicated by higher values)

	observational studies[1]	serious[1,2]	no serious inconsistency	no serious indirectness	serious	reporting bias[3]	325	–	–	–	⊕◯◯◯ VERY LOW	IMPORTANT
8												

sleep rate –279, 280······404 (follow – up 1 –3 months)

	observational studies[1]	serious[1,2]	no serious inconsistency	no serious indirectness	very serious	strong association[8]	181/2506 (7.2%)	–	–	–	⊕◯◯◯ VERY LOW	CRITICAL
47												

ineffect rate –277, 283······461 (follow – up 1 –4 months)

	observational studies[1]	serious[1,2]	no serious inconsistency	no serious indirectness	very serious	strong association[8]	273/3594 (7.6%)	–	–	–	⊕◯◯◯ VERY LOW	IMPORTANT
75												

ineffect rate (other criteria) –290, 291······587 (follow – up 0.5 –12 months)

	observational studies[1]	serious[1,2]	no serious inconsistency	no serious indirectness	very serious	very strong association[8]	1227/12629 (9.7%)	–	–	–	⊕◯◯◯ VERY LOW	NOT IMPORTANT
133												

1 case series.
2 RCTs failing to connect with authors.
3 the number of studies is small.
4 some authors are same or from the same unit.
5 the authors of these 2 duties are same.
6 the total number of cases is large.
7 a single study.
8 the total number of cases is large.

point injection for insomnia

Author (s):

Date: 2013 – 03 – 21

Question: Should point injection be used for insomnia?

Settings:

Bibliography:

| No of studies | Quality assessment | | | | | | No of patients | | Effect | | Quality | Importance |
	Design	Risk of bias	Inconsistency	Indirectness	Imprecision	Other considerations	Point injection	Control	Relative (95% CI)	Absolute		
PSQI – 251, 252 (range of scores: 0 – 21; Better indicated by lower values)												
2	observational studies[1]	serious[2]	no serious inconsistency	no serious indirectness	serious	reporting bias[3]	60	-	-	-	⊕○○○ VERY LOW	CRITICAL
sleep rate – 257												
1	observational studies[1]	serious[2]	no serious inconsistency	no serious indirectness	very serious[4]	reporting bias[5]	3/80 (3. 8%)	-	-	-	⊕○○○ VERY LOW	CRITICAL
sleep time (Better indicated by higher values)												
1	observational studies[1]	serious[2]	no serious inconsistency	no serious indirectness	serious	reporting bias[5]	29	-	-	-	⊕○○○ VERY LOW	IMPORTANT
ineffect rate – 251, 258 – 260 (follow – up 1 years)												
4	observational studies[1]	serious[1,2]	no serious inconsistency	no serious indirectness	serious	none	22/179 (12. 3%)	-	-	-	⊕○○○ VERY LOW	IMPORTANT
ineffect rate (other criteria) – 261 – 275 (follow – up 6 months)												
15	observational studies[1]	serious[1,2]	no serious inconsistency	no serious indirectness	very serious	none	51/1003 (5. 1%)	-	-	-	⊕○○○ VERY LOW	NOT IMPORTANT

1 case series.

2 RCTs failing to connect with the authors.

3 the number of studies is small.

4 No explanation was provided.

5 a single study.

roll acupuncture for insomnia

Author（s）：

Date：2013 – 03 – 19

Question：Should roll acupuncture be used for insomnia?

Settings：

Bibliography：

No of studies	Quality assessment						No of patients		Effect		Quality	Importance
	Design	Risk of bias	Inconsistency	Indirectness	Imprecision	Other considerations	Roll acupuncture	Control	Relative (95% CI)	Absolute		
PSQI – 194, 195 (follow – up mean 3 months; range of scores: 0 – 21; Better indicated by lower values)												
2	observational studies[1]	serious[2]	no serious inconsistency	no serious indirectness	serious	reporting bias[3]	180	-	-	-	⊕○○○ VERY LOW	CRITICAL
ineffect rate – 194, 195 (follow – up mean 3 months)												
2	observational studies[1]	serious[2]	no serious inconsistency	no serious indirectness	serious	reporting bias[3]	32/180 (17. 8%)	-	-	-	⊕○○○ VERY LOW	IMPORTANT

1 case series.

2 RCTs failing to connect with authors.

3 the number of studies is small, and the authors are the same.

scalp acupuncture for insomnia

Author（s）：

Date：2013 –03 –19

Question：Should scalp acupuncture be used for insomnia？

Settings：

Bibliography：

No of studies	Quality assessment						No of patients		Effect		Quality	Importance
	Design	Risk of bias	Inconsistency	Indirectness	Imprecision	Other considerations	Scalp acupuncture	Control	Relative (95% CI)	Absolute		
PSQI –211, 212 （range of scores: 0 –21; Better indicated by lower values）												
2	observational studies[1]	serious[2]	no serious inconsistency	no serious indirectness	serious	reporting bias[3]	112	-	-	-	⊕◯◯◯ VERY LOW	CRITICAL
ineffect rate –211, 212												
2	observational studies[1]	serious[2]	no serious inconsistency	no serious indirectness	very serious	reporting bias[3]	21/112 (18. 8%)	-	-	-	⊕◯◯◯ VERY LOW	IMPORTANT
clinical symotpms integrals –211 （range of scores: 0 –21; Better indicated by lower values）												
1	observational studies[1]	serious[2]	no serious inconsistency	no serious indirectness	serious	reporting bias[4]	32	-	-	-	⊕◯◯◯ VERY LOW	IMPORTANT
ineffect rate （other criteria） –213, 214 （follow –up mean 6 months）												
2	observational studies[1]	serious[1]	no serious inconsistency	no serious indirectness	very serious	reporting bias[3]	24/193 (12. 4%)	-	-	-	⊕◯◯◯ VERY LOW	NOT IMPORTANT

1 case series.

2 RCTs failing to connect with authors.

3 the number of studies is small.

4 a single study.

special acupuncture for insomnia

Author (s) :

Date: 2013 – 03 – 16

Question: Should special acupuncture be used for insomnia?

Settings:

Bibliography:

No of studies	Quality assessment						No of patients		Effect		Quality	Importance
	Design	Risk of bias	Inconsistency	Indirectness	Imprecision	Other considerations	Special acupuncture	Control	Relative (95% CI)	Absolute		
PSQI – penetrating needle – 16, 17 (measured with: PSQI scale; range of scores: 0 – 21; Better indicated by lower values)												
2	observational studies[1]	very serious[2]	no serious inconsistency	no serious indirectness	serious	reporting bias[3]	60	–	–	–	⊕◯◯◯ VERY LOW	CRITICAL
ineffect rate – penetrating needle – 16 – 19												
4	observational studies[1]	very serious[2]	no serious inconsistency	no serious indirectness	serious	reporting bias[3]	14/138 (10.1%)	–	–	–	⊕◯◯◯ VERY LOW	IMPORTANT
PSQI – abdominal acupuncture – 20 – 26 (follow – up 2 – 4 weeks; measured with: PSQI scale; range of scores: 0 – 3; Better indicated by lower values)												
7	observational studies[1]	very serious[4]	no serious inconsistency	no serious indirectness	very serious	reporting bias[5]	300	–	–	–	⊕◯◯◯ VERY LOW	CRITICAL
ineffect rate – abdominal acupuncture – 20, 21, 27 – 31 (follow – up 1 – 2 months)												
7	observational studies[1]	very serious[4]	no serious inconsistency	no serious indirectness	serious	none	22/256 (8.6%)	–	–	–	⊕◯◯◯ VERY LOW	IMPORTANT
SF – 36 – abdominal acupuncture – 24 (follow – up mean 2 weeks; range of scores: 0 – 100; Better indicated by higher values)												
1	observational studies[1]	very serious[6]	no serious inconsistency	no serious indirectness	very serious	reporting bias[3]	44	–	–	–	⊕◯◯◯ VERY LOW	NOT IMPORTANT

Continued

SPIEGEL – abdominal acupuncture – 33 (measured with: spiegel scale; range of scores: 0 – 7; Better indicated by lower values)

1	observational studies	serious	no serious inconsistency[7]	no serious indirectness	serious	reporting bias[3]	32	-	-	MD 14. 7 higher (0 to 10. 6 higher)	⊕◯◯◯ VERY LOW	NOT IMPORTANT

LSEQ – abdominal acupuncture – 32 (measured with: Leeds Sleep Evaluation Questionare; Better indicated by higher values)

1	observational studies[1]	very serious[6]	no serious inconsistency	no serious indirectness	serious	reporting bias[7]	36	-	-	-	⊕◯◯◯ VERY LOW	NOT IMPORTANT

SS – abdominal acupuncture – 34 (measured with: scores for symptoms; range of scores: 0 – 4; Better indicated by lower values)

1	observational studies	serious[8]	no serious inconsistency	no serious indirectness	serious	reporting bias[7]	40	-	-	MD 6.02 higher (0 to 1.25 higher)	⊕◯◯◯ VERY LOW	IMPORTANT

1 case series.
2 both of them are RCTs, but the authors can not be connected.
3 the number of studies is small.
4 they are case series or case reports, and RCTs failing to connect with authors.
5 the authors of 3 of them are same.
6 a RCT failing to connect author.
7 a singel study.
8 a before – after study and the disign is good.

sting therapyu for insomnia

Author (s):

Date: 2013 – 03 – 19

Question: Should bee sting therapyu be used for insomnia?

Settings:

Bibliography:

No of studies	Quality assessment						No of patients		Effect		Quality	Importance
	Design	Risk of bias	Inconsistency	Indirectness	Imprecision	Other considerations	Bee sting therapyu	Control	Relative (95% CI)	Absolute		
ineffect rate –229												
1	observational studies[1]	very serious[2]	no serious inconsistency	no serious indirectness	very serious	reporting bias[3]	2/41 (4.9%)	-	-	-	⊕○○○ VERY LOW	IMPORTANT
ineffect rate (other criteria) –230												
1	observational studies[1]	serious[1]	no serious inconsistency	no serious indirectness	very serious	reporting bias[3]	2/41 (4.9%)	-	-	-	⊕○○○ VERY LOW	NOT IMPORTANT

1 case series.

2 case series in the introduce of treatment experiences.

3 a single study.

thread or needle planting therapy for insomnia

Author（s）:

Date: 2013 – 03 – 20

Question: Should thread/needle planting therapy be used for insomnia?

Settings:

Bibliography:

| No of studies | Quality assessment | | | | | | No of patients | | Effect | | Quality | Importance |
	Design	Risk of bias	Inconsistency	Indirectness	Imprecision	Other considerations	Thread/needle planting therapy	Control	Relative (95% CI)	Absolute		
PSQI – 243 – 245（follow – up 1 – 12 months; range of scores: 0 – 21; Better indicated by lower values）												
3	observational studies[1]	serious[2]	no serious inconsistency	no serious indirectness	serious	reporting bias[3]	90	–	–	–	⊕◯◯◯ VERY LOW	CRITICAL
sleep rate – 243, 247												
2	observational studies[1]	serious[1]	no serious inconsistency	no serious indirectness	very serious	reporting bias[4]	4/82 (4.9%)	–	–	–	⊕◯◯◯ VERY LOW	CRITICAL
ineffect rate – 244, 245, 248（follow – up mean 1 months）												
3	observational studies[1]	serious[1,2]	no serious inconsistency	no serious indirectness	very serious	reporting bias[3]	14/144 (9.7%)	–	–	–	⊕◯◯◯ VERY LOW	IMPORTANT
ineffect rate – 249, 250												
2	observational studies[1]	serious[1]	no serious inconsistency	no serious indirectness	very serious	reporting bias[4]	4/51 (7.8%)	–	–	–	⊕◯◯◯ VERY LOW	NOT IMPORTANT

1 case series.

2 RCTs failing to connect with authors.

3 the number of studies is small, and 2 of them are from the same unit.

4 the number of studies is small.

warm needle moxibustion for insomnia

Author (s):

Date: 2013 – 03 – 20

Question: Should warm needle moxibustion be used for insomnia?

Settings:

Bibliography:

No of studies	Quality assessment						No of patients		Effect		Quality	Importance
	Design	Risk of bias	Inconsistency	Indirectness	Imprecision	Other considerations	Warm needle moxibustion	Control	Relative (95% CI)	Absolute		
AIS – 239 (range of scores: 0 – 48; Better indicated by lower values)												
1	observational studies[1]	serious[2]	no serious inconsistency	no serious indirectness	serious	reporting bias[3]	28	–	–	–	⊕○○○ VERY LOW	CRITICAL
sleep rate – 239, 240												
2	observational studies[1]	serious[1,2]	no serious inconsistency	no serious indirectness	very serious	reporting bias[4]	5/128 (3. 9%)	–	–	–	⊕○○○ VERY LOW	CRITICAL
ineffect rate (other criteria) – 241, 242												
2	observational studies[1]	serious[1]	no serious inconsistency	no serious indirectness	very serious	reporting bias[4]	4/77 (5. 2%)	–	–	–	⊕○○○ VERY LOW	NOT IMPORTANT

1 case series.

2 a RCT failing to connected with the author.

3 a single study.

4 the number of studies is small.

wrist – ankle needle for insomnia

Author (s) :

Date: 2013 – 03 – 20

Question: Should wrist – ankle needle be used for insomnia?

Settings:

Bibliography:

No of studies	Quality assessment						No of patients		Effect		Quality	Importance
	Design	Risk of bias	Inconsistency	Indirectness	Imprecision	Other considerations	Wrist – ankle needle	Control	Relative (95% CI)	Absolute		
ineffect rate (other criteria) – 236 – 238												
3	observational studies[1]	serious[1]	no serious inconsistency	no serious indirectness	very serious	reporting bias[2]	19/136 (14%)	–	–	–	⊕○○○ VERY LOW	NOT IMPORTANT

1 case series.

2 the number of studies is small.

acupuncture vs herb for insomnia

Author (s):

Date: 2012 - 04 - 09

Question: acupuncture vs herb for insomnia

Settings:

Bibliography: . acupuncture versus herb for insomnia. Cochrane Database of Systematic Reviews [Year], Issue [Issue].

No of studies	Quality assessment						No of patients		Effect		Quality	Importance
	Design	Risk of bias	Inconsistency	Indirectness	Imprecision	Other considerations	Acupuncture	Herb	Relative (95% CI)	Absolute		
ineffect rate												
1	randomised trials	serious[1]	no serious inconsistency	no serious indirectness	serious	reporting bias[2]	3/32 (9.4%)	OR 0.72 (0.15 to 3.53)		32 fewer per 1000 (from 104 fewer to 210 more)	⊕◯◯◯ VERY LOW	IMPORTANT
							4/32 (12.5%)			32 fewer per 1000 (from 104 fewer to 210 more)		
							12.5%					
PSQI (Better indicated by lower values)												
1	randomised trials	serious[1]	no serious inconsistency	no serious indirectness	serious	reporting bias[2]	32	–	MD 0.28 lower (0.67 lower to 0.11 higher)		⊕◯◯◯ VERY LOW	CRITICAL
							32					

1 there is no blinding method.

2 a single study.

acupuncture vs western medicine for insomnia

Author (s):

Date: 2012 –04 –09

Question: acupuncture vs western medicine for insomnia

Settings:

Bibliography: . acupuncture versus western medicine for insomnia. Cochrane Database of Systematic Reviews [Year] , Issue [Issue] .

No of studies	Quality assessment						No of patients		Effect		Quality	Importance
	Design	Risk of bias	Inconsistency	Indirectness	Imprecision	Other considerations	Acupuncture	Western medicine	Relative (95% CI)	Absolute		
spitzer (Better indicated by lower values)												
1	randomised trials	serious[1]	no serious inconsistency	no serious indirectness	no serious imprecision	reporting bias[2]	90	90	–	MD 0. 84 higher (0. 47 to 1. 21 higher)	⊕⊕○○ LOW	CRITICAL

1 there is no blinding method.

2 a single study.

acupuncture vs western medicine for insomnial

Author (s) :

Date: 2012 – 04 – 09

Question: acupuncture vs western medicine for insomnia

Settings:

Bibliography: . acupuncture versus western medicine for insomnia. Cochrane Database of Systematic Reviews [Year], Issue [Issue].

| No of studies | Quality assessment | | | | | | No of patients | | Effect | | Quality | Importance |
	Design	Risk of bias	Inconsistency	Indirectness	Imprecision	Other considerations	Acupuncture	Western medicine	Relative (95% CI)	Absolute		
ineffect rate												
4	randomised trials	serious[1,2]	no serious inconsistency	no serious indirectness	serious	reporting bias[3]	27/310 (8.7%)	78/200 (39%)	OR 0.16 (0.09 to 0.26)	297 fewer per 1000 (from 247 fewer to 336 fewer)	⊕◯◯◯ VERY LOW	IMPORTANT
							–	36.3%		279 fewer per 1000 (from 234 fewer to 314 fewer)		

1 allocation consealment: 2 of them are not so good.

2 there is no blinding method.

3 the number of studies is small.

special acupuncture vs normal acupuncture for insomnia

Author (s):

Date: 2012 – 04 – 09

Question: special acupuncture vs normal acupuncture for insomnia

Settings:

Bibliography: . special acupuncture versus normal acupuncture for insomnia. Cochrane Database of Systematic Reviews [Year], Issue [Issue] .

No of studies	Quality assessment						No of patients		Effect		Quality	Importance
	Design	Risk of bias	Inconsistency	Indirectness	Imprecision	Other considerations	Special acupuncture	Normal acupuncture	Relative (95% CI)	Absolute		

PSQI (Better indicated by lower values)

No of studies	Design	Risk of bias	Inconsistency	Indirectness	Imprecision	Other considerations	Special acupuncture	Normal acupuncture	Relative (95% CI)	Absolute	Quality	Importance
2	randomised trials	serious[1]	no serious inconsistency	no serious indirectness	no serious imprecision	reporting bias[2]	84	83	–	MD 2. 45 lower (3. 26 to 1. 64 lower)	⊕⊕◯◯ LOW	CRITICAL

ineffect

No of studies	Design	Risk of bias	Inconsistency	Indirectness	Imprecision	Other considerations	Special acupuncture	Normal acupuncture	Relative (95% CI)	Absolute	Quality	Importance
2	randomised trials	serious[3]	no serious inconsistency	no serious indirectness	serious	reporting bias[2]	7/68 (10. 3%)	18/64 (28. 1%)	OR 0.29 (0. 11 to 0.75)	179 fewer per 1000 (from 54 fewer to 240 fewer)	⊕◯◯◯ VERY LOW	IMPORTANT
							–	28. 7%		182 fewer per 1000 (from 55 fewer to 245 fewer)		

1 there is no blinding method in both studies.

2 the number of studies is small.

3 one study is connected with the professor who developed the abdominal acupuncture.

6 本《指南》推荐方案的形成过程
6.1 推荐方案初稿形成方法

首先，通过 Grade 评价等级的高低，依次推荐出治疗失眠的优势疗法（依次推荐了常规针刺、头穴透刺、耳穴、皮肤针、穴位注射五种疗法）。

其次，针对每一疗法进行具体方案的推荐时，该方案的主穴采用高质量文献主穴所使用的腧穴或穴组，配穴根据选用每一证型中使用频率最高的腧穴，操作方法、疗程采用高质量文献方案，注意事项综合文献及专家意见给出推荐。

6.2 针对推荐方案初稿的专家意见征询

将方案初稿形成专家意见征询问卷，分别向组内、组外专家征询意见，根据专家意见对初稿进行修改和调整（具体内容见附录8）。经过修改后的方案则为最终推荐方案。

7 本《指南》推荐方案征求意见稿
7.1 组内专家意见征集

失眠针灸临床实践指南初稿
专家意见征集表
（组内）

尊敬的专家您好：

对于您于百忙之中填写此份意见表，我们深表感谢。

请您协助本课题组完成以下三方面内容：

1. 请在表格的最后一列标明该方案是否推荐：

专家推荐同意原则：1 有效；2 安全；3 经济；4 操作便利；5 患者易接受；6 易普及；7 临床经验。

（例如：1 常规针刺法，如果您觉得可以推荐，则在最后一列画√，然后填原因2、6）

失眠循证针灸临床实践指南征求意见表

方案名称	方法		推荐级别	专家意见（同意√不同意×）
	病情	概述：如选穴、手法/方法/操作、疗程		
1 常规针刺法	一般人群	推荐脏腑辨证基础上的常规针刺法 ①主穴：神门、四神聪、三阴交 ②配穴：风池、太阳、本神 ③辨证（均双侧取穴）：肝火上扰型配太冲、肝俞、行间；肝郁脾虚型配神门、太冲、足三里；心脾两虚型配心俞、脾俞；心胆气虚型配心俞、胆俞、丘墟；心火炽盛型配心俞、肾俞、太溪、郄门；气滞血瘀型配太冲、血海、气海、肝俞、心俞	B 级	
2 头穴透刺法	一般人群	建议头部安神腧穴透刺法为主，兼顾脏腑辨证 ①主穴：前神聪透神庭、左右头临泣透左右神聪、后神聪透强间 ②配穴：络却透通天、承光透曲差	B 级	

方案名称	方法		推荐级别	专家意见（同意√不同意×）
	病情	概述：如选穴、手法/方法/操作、疗程		
3 耳穴压丸法	一般人群	慢性失眠建议耳穴压丸法作为常规针刺法的补充疗法；短期或轻度失眠建议单独使用 ①主穴：神门、皮质下、交感、内分泌、枕 ②配穴：心、肾 ③辨证：心脾两虚型配脾、心、胃；阴虚火旺型配肾、肝；胃腑不和型配胃、脾；肝郁化火型配肝、胆	C 级	
4 皮肤针法	一般人群	建议膀胱经及督脉皮肤针法，也可作为针刺的配合疗法 ①取穴：背部足太阳膀胱经一、二侧线及督脉为主 ②操作方法：a. 皮肤针：患者俯卧位，沿膀胱经第一、二侧线由上向下，督脉由下向上进行叩击，每次叩击之间距离为 0.5cm，反复叩击 5 分钟，以皮肤潮红为度，膀胱经第一、二侧线实证可叩至皮肤微出血；b. 滚针：患者俯卧位，针具从背部足太阳膀胱经第一侧线由上而下滚动，督脉由下而上顺经脉循行滚动，以较慢速度循经滚动 10 次左右，用力大小因人而异，以患者感到舒适、皮肤红润为度	C 级	
5 穴位注射法	一般人群（顽固性失眠）	顽固性失眠建议配合维生素 B_{12} 注射液穴位注射 ①取穴：风池、心俞 ②药物：维生素 B_{12} 注射液 ③操作方法：在上述腧穴注射，局部出现酸、麻、胀或放射感后，回抽，如无回血则可缓慢注入维生素 B_{12} 注射液，每穴 0.1mg，左右穴交替	C 级	

2. 请给您认为可以推荐的方案排序（请按照降序排列）：

3. 请您留下其他相关意见（如您认为值得推荐但未推荐的方案，推荐方案中还有那些需要改进之处等）：

最后请您留下您的专业信息：

姓名：

职称：　　　　　　　　　　　　　　　　专业：

再次感谢您的配合，谢谢！

针灸临床实践指南失眠组

2013 年 6 月 9 日

7.2 组外专家意见征集

失眠针灸临床实践指南初稿
专家意见征集表
（组外）

尊敬的专家您好：

首先，对于您抽出宝贵时间阅读并回答本问卷，我们深表感谢！

本课题"失眠针灸临床实践指南"，以 GRADE 体系为基本评价工具（GRADE 为系统评价和指南提供了一个证据质量评价体系，同时也为指南中的推荐强度评价提供了一种系统方法），以证据质量、利弊平衡、价值观和意愿、资源消耗与成本分析为关键因素，通过对目前文献的评价和权衡，初步形成"失眠针灸临床实践指南初稿"。

本次问卷调查，旨在依据您的临床实践经验，对本课题形成的"失眠针灸临床实践指南初稿"给予宝贵意见，以为我们下一步的工作提供重要依据。本问卷由两部分组成（一是对具体方案的推荐意见，二是对方案的排序），请您尽可能填写完整。谢谢！

形成推荐意见的关键因素

	1. 证据质量是依据 GRADE 证据体系得出的评价结果
	2. 影响证据质量等级的方面主要有 5 个：试验设计、试验结果的一致性、是否存在间接的比较、精确度及是否存在发表偏倚
证据质量	3. 证据质量分为高（A）、中（B）、低（C）、极低（D）四个等级：①证据质量高表示未来研究几乎不可能改变现有疗效评价结果的可信度；②证据质量中表示未来研究可能对现有疗效评估有重要影响，可能改变评价结果的可信度；③证据质量低表示未来研究很有可能对现有疗效评价有重要影响，改变评估结果可信度的可能性较大；④证据质量极低表示任何疗效评估都很不确定
	4. 证据质量越高越有利于推荐
利弊平衡	利弊间的差别越大，越合适强推荐；差别越小，越合适弱推荐即利越大，弊越小，越容易作出推荐
意愿价值观	患者意愿价值观越一致，越容易作出推荐
资源成本分析	一项干预措施的花费越高，即消耗的资源越多，越不适合强推荐

推荐等级描述方法

GRADE 推荐强度采用数字 1、2 描述，文献质量等级用 A、B、C、D 描述。例如：GRADE 1C 为强推荐，低质量证据；GRADE 2D 为弱推荐，极低质量证据。

鉴于课题研究的需要，非常希望您能首先配合回答以下问题：

您的年龄：＿＿＿＿＿＿＿　　　　您的职称：＿＿＿＿＿＿＿

您的学历：＿＿＿＿＿＿＿　　　　您所在医院的级别：＿＿＿＿＿＿＿＿＿

您从事针灸临床工作的时间＿＿＿＿＿＿＿年

您是否了解 GRADE 方法：　　　　了解□　　　　不了解□

您是否听说过 GRADE 方法：　　　　　　　听说过□　　没听说过□

您是否了解临床指南制作流程：　　　　　　了解□　　　不了解□

您对本问卷作答是基于（可多选）：　　　　临床经验□　专业知识□　　　科研经历□

为方便进一步方案修改时专家意见的征集，请您留下联系方式（自愿选择，我们承诺对相关信息的保密）：

您的姓名：_____

您的工作单位：_____

您的 E－mail：_____

注：为便于电子版操作，问卷中需要画钩的选项用黄色标示即可，例如：

您是否了解 GRADE 方法：　　　了解□　　　　　　　不了解□

第一部分：具体方案推荐意见

方案 1	项目	内容	您是否推荐			不推荐原因
常规毫针刺法	治疗原则	辨证施治，兼以安神	推荐	强推荐□ 弱推荐□	不推荐□	原因：
	取穴	①主穴：神门、四神聪、三阴交 ②配穴：风池、太阳、本神 ③辨证（均双侧取穴）：肝火上扰型配太冲、肝俞、行间；肝郁脾虚型配太冲、足三里；心脾两虚型配心俞、脾俞；心胆气虚型配心俞、胆俞、丘墟；心火炽盛型配心俞、肾俞、太溪、郄门；气滞血瘀型配太冲、血海、气海、肝俞、心俞	推荐	强推荐□ 弱推荐□	不推荐□	原因：
	操作方法	四神聪平刺，针尖方向均朝向百会方向，本神平刺，其余腧穴均采用常规针刺法，针刺得气后，主、配穴均使用平补平泻法，辨证取穴根据证型行相应补泻手法，行针 1 分钟后留针	推荐	强推荐□ 弱推荐□	不推荐□	原因：
	疗程	每次留针 30 分钟，每周 5 次，10 次为 1 个疗程	推荐	强推荐□ 弱推荐□	不推荐□	原因：
	注意事项	临床应用时可于主穴适当配合使用电针（疏波）	推荐	强推荐□ 弱推荐□	不推荐□	原因：

推荐意见：失眠推荐脏腑辨证基础上的常规针刺法

GRADE 1B

推荐强度：1　证据等级：B

您是否推荐常规针刺法治疗方案

推　荐：强推荐□　　　　　不推荐□　　　　　　不推荐原因：
　　　　弱推荐□

方案 2	项目	内容	您是否推荐			不推荐原因
头穴透刺法	治疗原则	疏通脑络，镇静安神	推荐	强推荐□ 弱推荐□	不推荐□	原因：
	取穴	①主穴：前神聪透神庭、左右头临泣透左右神聪、后神聪透强间 ②配穴：络却透通天、承光透曲差	推荐	强推荐□ 弱推荐□	不推荐□	原因：
	操作方法	①针刺方向：由前神聪进针，平刺透向神庭；由头临泣进针，平刺透向同侧神聪；由后神聪进针，平刺透向强间 ②具体操作：采用（0.35～0.40）mm×（40～50）mm 毫针，针身与头皮呈 15°角，快速刺入头皮下，当针尖到达帽状腱膜下层，指下感到阻力减小时，将针与头皮平行，继续捻转进针，各穴进针深度为 30～40mm，然后快速小幅度左右捻针，每针行针约 1 分钟，取得较强针感后留针	推荐	强推荐□ 弱推荐□	不推荐□	原因：
	疗程	每次留针 30 分钟，每天 1 次，5 次为 1 个疗程，疗程之间间隔 2 天	推荐	强推荐□ 弱推荐□	不推荐□	原因：
	注意事项	临床应用时，头穴透刺作为主要治疗方法，需同时根据患者病情，辨证加用其他腧穴，针刺方法采用常规刺法	推荐	强推荐□ 弱推荐□	不推荐□	原因：

推荐意见：失眠建议头部安神腧穴透刺法为主，兼顾脏腑辨证

GRADE 2D

推荐强度：2 证据等级：D

您是否推荐头穴透刺法治疗方案

推　荐：强推荐□　　　　　　不推荐□　　　　　不推荐原因：
　　　　弱推荐□

方案3	项目	内容	您是否推荐		不推荐原因
耳穴 贴压法	治疗原则	扶阴抑阳，镇静安神	推荐	强推荐□ 弱推荐□	不推荐□	原因：
	取穴	①主穴：神门、皮质下、交感、内分泌、枕 ②配穴：心、肾 ③辨证：心脾两虚型配脾、心、胃；阴虚火旺型配肾、肝；胃腑不和型配胃、脾；肝郁化火型配肝、胆	推荐	强推荐□ 弱推荐□	不推荐□	原因：
	操作方法	针刺结束后，将王不留行籽（或磁珠）贴于0.5cm×0.5cm的医用胶布中央，耳穴常规消毒后，将粘有王不留行籽（或磁珠）的胶布贴在以上耳穴，并适度按压，使耳穴有胀、热、微痛感，每晚睡前按1次，约5分钟，以耳郭微红、微热为度，隔天换贴1次，双耳交替操作	推荐	强推荐□ 弱推荐□	不推荐□	原因：
	疗程	常规针灸治疗后进行，每3天更换1次，4次为1个疗程	推荐	强推荐□ 弱推荐□	不推荐□	原因：
	注意事项	耳穴压丸疗法一般作为常规针刺法的延续治疗方法，单独使用疗效有限；只有短期或者轻度失眠患者单独使用可获较满意疗效	推荐	强推荐□ 弱推荐□	不推荐□	原因：

推荐意见：慢性失眠建议耳穴压丸法作为常规针刺法的补充疗法；短期或轻度失眠建议单独使用

GRADE 2D

推荐强度：2 证据等级：D

您是否推荐耳穴压丸法治疗方案

推　荐：强推荐□　　　　　　　不推荐□　　　　　　不推荐原因：
　　　　弱推荐□

方案4	项目	内容	您是否推荐			不推荐原因
皮肤针法	治疗原则	调整脏腑，通督安神	推荐	强推荐□ 弱推荐□	不推荐□	原因：
	取穴	背部足太阳膀胱经一、二侧线及督脉为主	推荐	强推荐□ 弱推荐□	不推荐□	原因：
	操作方法	皮肤针：患者俯卧位，沿膀胱经第一、二侧线由上向下，督脉由下向上进行叩击，每次叩击之间距离为0.5cm，反复叩击5分钟，以皮肤潮红为度，膀胱经第一、二侧线实证可叩至皮肤微出血	推荐	强推荐□ 弱推荐□	不推荐□	原因：
		滚针：患者俯卧位，针具从背部足太阳膀胱经第一侧线由上而下滚动，督脉由下而上顺经脉循行滚动，以较慢速度循经滚动10次左右，用力大小因人而异，以患者感到舒适、皮肤红润为度	推荐	强推荐□ 弱推荐□	不推荐□	原因：
	疗程	每次治疗15～20分钟，隔天1次，10次为1个疗程	推荐	强推荐□ 弱推荐□	不推荐□	原因：
	注意事项	如叩刺出血，嘱患者24小时针孔避水，防止感染（此疗法可单独使用，也可作为针刺的配合疗法）	推荐	强推荐□ 弱推荐□	不推荐□	原因：

推荐意见：失眠建议膀胱经及督脉皮肤针法；也可作为针刺的配合疗法

GRADE 2D

推荐强度：2　证据等级：D

您是否推荐皮肤针法治疗方案

推　荐：强推荐□　　　　　不推荐□　　　　　不推荐原因：
　　　　弱推荐□

注：在组内意见征询中，有专家建议将"操作方法"中的"滚针"去掉，无论您是否推荐，请均给出原因，谢谢

续表

方案5	项目	内容	您是否推荐			不推荐原因
穴位注射法	治疗原则	宁心安神	推荐	强推荐□ 弱推荐□	不推荐□	原因：
	取穴	风池、心俞	推荐	强推荐□ 弱推荐□	不推荐□	原因：
	药物	维生素 B_{12} 注射液	推荐	强推荐□ 弱推荐□	不推荐□	原因：
	操作方法	在上述腧穴注射，局部出现酸、麻、胀或放射感后，回抽，如无回血则可缓慢注入维生素 B_{12} 注射液，每穴 0.1mg，左右穴交替操作	推荐	强推荐□ 弱推荐□	不推荐□	原因：
	疗程	每天 1 次，左右穴交替，10 次为 1 个疗程	推荐	强推荐□ 弱推荐□	不推荐□	原因：
	注意事项	穴位注射当天局部避水，避免热敷；注射局部吸收不良时，可待吸收完全后再行治疗	推荐	强推荐□ 弱推荐□	不推荐□	原因：

推荐意见：顽固失眠建议配合维生素 B_{12} 注射液穴位注射

GRADE 2D

推荐强度：2 证据等级：D

您是否推荐穴位注射法治疗方案

推　荐：强推荐□　　　　　　　不推荐□　　　　　　不推荐原因：
　　　　弱推荐□

第二部分：方案排序

请根据您的临床经验及相关知识，对上述方案进行推荐排序：_____

1　常规针刺法
2　头穴透刺法
3　耳穴压丸法
4　皮肤针法
5　穴位注射法

此外，如果您对该指南推荐方案还有其他意见或建议，请写在这里：

最后，对于您的协助，我们再次表示衷心感谢，对于您的宝贵意见，我们将在临床实践指南中予以体现。谢谢！

失眠临床实践指南课题组

2013 年 8 月 19 日

8 专家意见征集过程、结果汇总及处理

8.1 组内专家意见征询结果

以发放问卷的方式进行，共发出问卷 25 份，回收 7 份。

8.1.1 专家基本情况

均为高级职称临床人员，其中正高占 71.5%，副高占 28.6%。

8.1.2 通过率

常规针刺法：100%（7/7）

头穴透刺法：71.4%（5/7）

耳穴压丸法：100%（7/7）

皮肤针法：71.4%（5/7））

穴位注射法：85.7%（6/7）

结果：所有方案均通过。

8.1.3 排序（按照排序高低，分别赋予 5 至 1 分）

常规针刺法：35

头穴透刺法：15

耳穴压丸法：24

皮肤针法：14

穴位注射法：8

结果：通过的方案中，专家意见推荐顺序为常规针刺、耳穴压丸、头穴透刺、皮肤针、穴位注射。

8.1.4 其他意见

瘀瘀较重患者可以考虑放血；穴位注射穴位是否为最佳选择；常规针刺中，辨证分型是否考虑痰火扰心型；滚针不清楚，且临床应用较少，建议去除此部分。

8.2 组外专家意见征询结果

以发放问卷的方式进行，共发出问卷 54 份，回收 14 份。

8.2.1 专家基本情况

均为高级职称临床人员，其中正高占 85.7%，副高占 14.3%。

均为本科以上学历，其中博士以上占 50%。

三甲医院从业占 71.4%，针灸专科医院从业占 28.6%。

平均年龄 48.7 岁，平均工作时间 24.5 年。

8.2.2 通过率

8.2.2.1 常规针刺法

通过率为 100%（强推荐 85.7%，弱推荐 14.3%，有 2 位专家提出此处治疗原则需要修改，有 2 位专家建议修改取穴）。

8.2.2.2 头穴透刺法

通过率为 85.7%（强推荐 50%，弱推荐 25.7%）。

8.2.2.3 耳穴压丸法

通过率为 100%（强推荐 42.9%，弱推荐 57.1%，有 1 位专家提出治疗原则需要修改）。

8.2.2.4 皮肤针法

通过率为 71.4%（弱推荐 71.4%，有 71.4% 的专家建议去掉滚针，原因为临床使用不普遍）。

8.2.2.5 穴位注射法

通过率为 54.1%（弱推荐 54.1%，原因包括疗效不稳定、患者接受度差、护理不便）。

结果：所有方案均通，但皮肤针法中的滚针未获通过。根据通过率，需要调整头穴透刺法和耳穴压丸法的推荐顺序。

8.2.3 排序（按照排序高低，分别赋予5至1分）

常规针刺法：69

头穴透刺法：41

耳穴压丸法：45

皮肤针法：27

穴位注射法：16

结果：通过的方案中，专家意见推荐顺序为常规针刺、耳穴压丸、头穴透刺、皮肤针、穴位注射。

8.3 推荐方案

根据上述意见，将专家未达成共识的内容——滚针去掉，同时调整头穴透刺法和耳穴压丸法的推荐顺序。另外，对于达到一级共识，且专家推荐力度较大的耳穴压丸法和头穴透刺法的证据级别提升一级，形成推荐方案。

8.3.1 毫针刺法

毫针刺法是针灸疗法的基本针刺方法，应用最为广泛，具有灵活性强的特点。毫针刺法是建立在中医辨证论治的基础上，根据患者证型进行针对性治疗。由于掌握了患者的整体情况和疾病特点，因而能标本兼治，从而起效。其疗效优于西药，与中药持平。

治疗原则：辨证施治，兼以安神。

取穴：①主穴：神门、四神聪、三阴交。②配穴：风池、太阳、本神。

辨证（均双侧取穴）：肝火上扰型配太冲、肝俞、行间；肝郁脾虚型配太冲、足三里；心脾两虚型配心俞、脾俞；心胆气虚型配心俞、胆俞、丘墟；心火炽盛型配心俞、肾俞、太溪、郄门；气滞血瘀型配太冲、血海、气海、肝俞、心俞。

操作方法：四神聪平刺，针尖方向均朝向百会；本神平刺。其余腧穴均采用常规针刺法。针刺得气后，主、配穴均使用平补平泻法，辨证取穴根据证型行相应补泻手法，行针1分钟后留针。

疗程：每次留针30分钟，每周5次，10次为1个疗程。

注意事项：临床应用时可于主穴适当配合使用电针（疏波）。

『推荐』

> 失眠推荐脏腑辨证基础上的毫针刺法。［GRADE 1B］

8.3.2 耳穴压丸法

耳穴压丸疗法是通过针刺、压豆等方法刺激耳郭穴位来治疗疾病的一种疗法。此疗法本身具有平衡大脑皮层的兴奋与抑制，从而使皮层功能活动趋于正常的作用。在失眠的治疗中，常规针刺结束后采用耳穴压丸的方式，在补充针灸治疗的基础上，更能给予大脑皮层持久的小剂量刺激，更符合失眠的疾病特点，故而配合使用，长期疗效可靠。

治疗原则：镇静安神。

取穴：①主穴：神门、皮质下、交感、内分泌、枕。②配穴：心、肾。

辨证：心脾两虚型配脾、心、胃；阴虚火旺型配肾、肝；胃腑不和型配胃、脾；肝郁化火型配肝、胆。

操作方法：针刺结束后，将王不留行籽（或磁珠）贴于0.5cm×0.5cm的医用胶布中央，耳穴常规消毒后，将粘有王不留行籽（或磁珠）的胶布贴在以上耳穴，并适度按压，使耳穴有胀、热、微痛感，每晚睡前按1次，约5分钟，以耳郭微红、微热为度，隔天换贴1次，双耳交替操作。

疗程：常规针灸治疗后进行，每3天更换1次，4次为1个疗程。

注意事项：耳穴压丸疗法一般作为毫针刺法的延续治疗方法，单独使用疗效有限；只有短期或者轻度失眠患者单独使用可获较满意疗效。

『推荐』

> 慢性失眠建议耳穴压丸法作为毫针刺法的补充疗法；短期或轻度失眠建议单独使用。[GRADE 2C]

8.3.3　头穴透刺法

透刺法是指将毫针刺入腧穴后，按一定方向刺向另一（几）个腧穴的一种刺法，多是平刺或斜刺的延伸应用。透刺法是通经行气、增强刺激的一种重要手法，将此针刺方法应用到头部相应腧穴，在增强腧穴本身镇静安神作用的同时，可以有效疏通头部郁阻的经脉，从而取得理想的疗效。临床研究表明，其疗效优于常规针刺法。

治疗原则：疏通脑络，镇静安神。

取穴：①主穴：前神聪透神庭、左右头临泣透左右神聪、后神聪透强间。②配穴：络却透通天、承光透曲差。

操作方法：针刺方向，由前神聪进针，平刺透向神庭；由头临泣进针，平刺透向同侧神聪；由后神聪进针，平刺透向强间。采用直径0.35～0.40mm、长度40～50mm的毫针，针身与头皮呈15°角，快速刺入头皮下，当针尖到达帽状腱膜下层，指下感到阻力减小时，将针与头皮平行，继续捻转进针，各穴进针深度为1～1.5寸，然后快速小幅度左右捻针，每针行针约1分钟，取得较强针感后留针。

疗程：每次留针30分钟，每天1次，5次为1个疗程，疗程之间间隔2天。

注意事项：临床应用时，头穴透刺作为主要治疗方法，需同时根据患者病情，辨证加用其他腧穴，针刺方法采用常规刺法。

『推荐』

> 失眠建议头部安神腧穴透刺法为主，兼顾脏腑辨证。[GRADE 2C]

8.3.4　皮肤针法

皮肤针法是利用皮肤针（梅花针）刺激十二皮部，从而激发经气、治疗疾病的一种疗法。运用皮肤针治疗失眠，主要通过刺激膀胱经第一侧线及督脉来达到调整脏腑功能、疏达任督脉气的作用，从而使"脏腑调而神气安"。该疗法单独使用时疗效与西药相当[50]，但是优势在于不产生耐药性及不良反应。

治疗原则：调整脏腑，通督安神。

取穴：背部足太阳膀胱经第一、二侧线及督脉为主。

操作方法：选用皮肤针治疗。患者俯卧位，沿膀胱经第一、二侧线由上向下，督脉由下向上进行叩击，每次叩击之间距离为0.5cm，反复叩击5分钟，以皮肤潮红为度。膀胱经第一、二侧线实证可叩至皮肤微出血。

疗程：每次治疗15～20分钟，隔天1次，10次为1个疗程。

注意事项：如叩刺出血，嘱患者24小时针孔避水，防止感染（此疗法可单独使用，也可作为针刺的配合疗法）。

『推荐』

> 失眠建议采用膀胱经及督脉皮肤针疗法；也可作为针刺的配合疗法。[GRADE 2D]

8.3.5 穴位注射法

穴位注射是将药物注入腧穴以防治疾病的一种疗法，它将针刺、药理、药水对腧穴的渗透刺激作用结合在一起发挥综合效果，对于某些顽固性疾病效果可靠。主要用作顽固性失眠的辅助疗法。但目前尚无有力证据证明其与其他疗法在疗效方面的优劣关系。

治疗原则：宁心安神。

取穴：风池、心俞。

药物：维生素 B_{12} 注射液。

操作方法：在上述腧穴注射，局部出现酸、麻、胀或放射感后，回抽，如无回血则可缓慢注入维生素 B_{12} 注射液，每穴 0.1mg。左右穴交替操作。

疗程：每天 1 次，左右穴交替，10 次为 1 个疗程。

注意事项：穴位注射当天局部避水，避免热敷；注射局部吸收不良时，可待吸收完全后再行治疗。

『推荐』

> 顽固失眠建议配合维生素 B_{12} 注射液穴位注射。［GRADE 2D］

8.4 专家审查会意见

意见汇总处理表

序号	指南章条编号	意见内容	处理意见	备注
1	针灸治疗和推荐方案5	推荐意见中并未阐明推荐理由，未阐明推荐方案能解决什么临床具体问题	已按照专家意见修改	
2	诊断标准2；针灸治疗和推荐方案2、5	去掉新药使用的指导方案，强调治疗方法的针对性，不建议依据中药新药临床指导原则	已按照专家意见修改	此次进行进一步修改
3	针灸治疗和推荐方案5	应介绍每个治疗方案在什么情况下应用	已按照专家意见修改	
4	针灸治疗和推荐方案3、4	健康教育是针灸医生不可忽视的，与临床疗效密切相关的因素	已按照专家意见修改	按照此次专家意见，将"注意事项"和"健康教育"部分都进行了修改
5	针灸治疗和推荐方案5.1	取穴原则、治疗原则方面的语言调整	已按照专家意见修改	
6	针灸治疗和推荐方案5	"安眠穴"推荐为主穴；照海、申脉的应用；顽固性失眠不建议穴位注射；头穴透刺法要明确其疗效特点，如起效快	未采纳	5.7未采纳，主要因为目前尚没有足够的证据，所以在本指南中暂未予以推荐/不推荐，课题组考虑将此意见纳入第一次指南更新的过程中，如果在更新前有新的临床证据出现，我们可以补充推荐
7	针灸治疗和推荐方案5	穴位埋线疗法是治疗失眠的有效方法，建议纳入	未采纳	

序号	指南章条编号	意见内容	处理意见	备注
8	针灸治疗和推荐方案 5.1	出现频次高的腧穴间相配是否就是最优	未采纳	关于腧穴配伍与腧穴运用频次之间的关系问题,课题组是在分析腧穴处方组成结构和还原处方结构的基础上,取每一部分中临床运用最多的穴组进行推荐的,所以综合考虑了临床运用的实际
9	针灸治疗和推荐方案 1、5.1	1 中,"特点"内容未及,宜补,"原则"稍笼统;5.1 中,"毫针的疗效优于西药",此处下结论应慎重	已按照专家意见修改	
10	针灸治疗和推荐方案 5.1	建议使用针灸临床实际辨证取穴,避免套用中医临床诊断分型	部分采纳	在推荐辨证分型时,课题组是根据临床报道中最常见的证型进行推荐的,所以综合考虑了临床运用的实际
11	针灸治疗和推荐方案 5	缺少特征性分析,需要指出治疗特点	已根据专家意见修改	根据每一种疗法中关键结局指标重点指向的问题进行了分析,在推荐方案中,对每一种疗法能够具体解决的问题,或者针对的某一特定人群进行了标示
12	诊断标准	观察诊断的客观评价,可使用一些量表,建议主客观观察结合	未采纳	各种失眠量表主要用于疗效的判定,也就是本研究中各种"关键结局指标"(常用的匹兹堡指数、阿森斯睡眠量表等在本研究中均有应用),但在中西医诊断标准中,少有以量表为标准者,所以课题组暂未采纳
13	诊断标准 2	中医诊断标准及分型是 1994 年制定的标准,是否有更新		此标准目前尚无更新版本
14	其他	语言应规范、严谨,应使用标准用词,如"应、可、宜",如推荐方案,宜用"可推荐",而不宜用"建议推荐"	部分采纳	
15	其他	各种方法的概述应删除,不应给予定义式描述	部分采纳	

根据专家审查会意见,将推荐方案进行以下调整。

8.4.1 毫针刺法

毫针刺法是针灸疗法的基本针刺方法,临床应用最为广泛,同时具有灵活性强的特点。由于掌握了患者的整体情况和疾病特点,毫针刺法在改善失眠患者整体睡眠质量方面(包括睡眠质量、入睡时间、睡眠时间、睡眠效率、睡眠障碍、催眠药物应用、日间功能障碍)效果显著,尤其在改善患者日间觉醒状态方面疗效突出。有研究表明，毫针刺法的疗效可优于某些西药[34－37]，也可达到与中草药相当[38]的效果。

治疗原则：安神定志，辨证取穴。

取穴：①主穴：神门、四神聪、三阴交。②配穴：风池、太阳、本神。

辨证（均双侧取穴）：肝郁化火型配太冲、肝俞、行间；肝郁痰扰型配太冲、足三里；心脾两虚型配心俞、脾俞；心虚胆怯型配心俞、胆俞、丘墟；阴虚火旺型配心俞、肾俞、太溪、郄门；气滞血瘀型配太冲、血海、气海、肝俞、心俞。

操作方法：四神聪平刺，针尖方向朝向百会；本神向后平刺。其余腧穴均采用常规针刺法。针刺得气后，主、配穴均使用平补平泻法，辨证取穴根据证型行相应补泻手法，行针1分钟后留针。

疗程：每次留针30分钟，每周5次，10次为1个疗程。

注意事项：临床应用时可于主穴适当配合使用电针（疏波）。

『推荐』

> 在改善失眠患者整体睡眠质量，尤其是日间觉醒状态方面，推荐使用结合脏腑辨证的毫针刺法。［GRADE 1B］

8.4.2 耳穴压丸法

耳穴压丸疗法能够平衡大脑皮层的兴奋与抑制，从而使皮层的功能活动趋于正常。因此，其疗效主要体现在改善患者睡眠时间、睡眠质量方面，其对于睡眠其他方面的改善尚少有研究。另外，在失眠治疗中，常规针刺结束后采用耳穴压丸的方式，在补充针灸治疗的基础上，更能给予皮层持久的小剂量刺激，更符合失眠的疾病特点。

治疗原则：镇静安神。

取穴：①主穴：神门、皮质下、交感、内分泌、枕。②配穴：心、肾。

辨证：心脾两虚型配脾、心、胃；阴虚火旺型配肾、肝；胃腑不和型配胃、脾；肝郁化火型配肝、胆。

操作方法：针刺结束后，将王不留行籽（或磁珠）贴于0.5cm×0.5cm的医用胶布中央，耳穴常规消毒后，将粘有王不留行籽（或磁珠）的胶布贴在以上耳穴，并适度按压，使耳穴有胀、热、微痛感，每晚睡前按1次，约5分钟，以耳郭微红、微热为度，隔天换贴1次，双耳交替操作。

疗程：常规针灸治疗后进行，每3天更换1次，4次为1个疗程。

注意事项：耳穴压丸疗法一般作为毫针刺法的延续治疗方法，单独使用疗效有限；只有短期或者轻度失眠患者单独使用可获较满意疗效。

『推荐』

> 在改善失眠患者睡眠时间和睡眠质量方面，建议使用耳穴压丸法。其中，慢性失眠建议将其作为毫针刺法的补充疗法；急性或亚急性失眠建议单独使用。［GRADE 2C］

8.4.3 头穴透刺法

透刺法作为平刺或斜刺的延伸应用，是通经行气、增强刺激的一种重要手法。将其应用于头部腧穴，在增强腧穴本身镇静安神作用的同时，可以有效疏通头部郁阻的经脉，因此更适用于伴有日间功能障碍的失眠患者，在改善其睡眠时间和睡眠质量的同时，可以有效提高日间活动效率。相关研究表明其疗效可优于毫针刺法[39]。

治疗原则：疏通脑络，镇静安神。

取穴：①主穴：前神聪透神庭、左右头临泣透左右神聪、后神聪透强间。②配穴：络却透通天、承光透曲差。

操作方法：针刺方向，由前神聪进针，平刺透向神庭；由头临泣进针，平刺透向同侧神聪；由后神聪进针，平刺透向强间。采用直径 0.35～0.40mm、长度 40～50mm 的毫针，针身与头皮呈 15°角，快速刺入头皮下，当针尖到达帽状腱膜下层，指下感到阻力减小时，将针与头皮平行，继续捻转进针，各穴进针深度为 1～1.5 寸，然后快速小幅度左右捻针，每针行针约 1 分钟，取得较强针感后留针。

疗程：每次留针 30 分钟，每天 1 次，5 次为 1 个疗程，疗程之间间隔 2 天。

注意事项：临床应用时，头穴透刺作为主要治疗方法，需同时根据患者病情，辨证加用其他腧穴，针刺方法采用常规刺法。

『推荐』

> 伴有日间功能障碍的失眠患者，建议使用以头部安神腧穴透刺法为主，兼顾脏腑辨证的针刺疗法。［GRADE 2C］

8.4.4 皮肤针法

皮肤针法主要通过刺激十二皮部产生治疗作用，因刺激部位浅，刺激量相对较轻，而易被患者尤其是敏感人群接受，应用范围广泛。运用皮肤针治疗失眠，主要通过刺激膀胱经第一侧线及督脉来达到调整脏腑功能、疏达任督脉气的作用，除了能有效改善睡眠质量外，还能有效缩短患者入睡时间。研究表明，本疗法单独使用时可达到与某些西药相当的疗效[36]。此疗法突出优势在于不易产生耐药性及不良反应。

治疗原则：调整脏腑，通督安神。

取穴：背部足太阳膀胱经第一、二侧线及督脉为主。

操作方法：采用皮肤针治疗。患者俯卧位，沿膀胱经第一、二侧线由上向下，督脉由下向上进行叩击，每次叩击之间距离为 0.5cm，反复叩击 5 分钟，以皮肤潮红为度。膀胱经第一、二侧线实证可叩至皮肤微出血。

疗程：每次治疗 15～20 分钟，隔天 1 次，10 次为 1 个疗程。

注意事项：如叩刺出血，嘱患者 24 小时针孔避水，防止感染（此疗法可单独使用，也可作为针刺的配合疗法）。

『推荐』

> 在改善失眠患者入睡困难方面，建议使用膀胱经及督脉皮肤针疗法；也可作为毫针刺法的配合疗法。［GRADE 2D］

8.4.5 穴位注射法

穴位注射是将药物注入腧穴以防治疾病的一种疗法，它将针刺、药理、药水对腧穴的渗透刺激作用结合在一起发挥综合效果，对于某些顽固性疾病效果可靠。主要用作顽固性失眠的辅助疗法。但目前尚无有力证据证明其与其他疗法在疗效方面的优劣关系。

治疗原则：疏通脑络，宁心安神。

取穴：风池、心俞。

药物：维生素 B_{12} 注射液。

操作方法：在上述腧穴注射，局部出现酸、麻、胀或放射感后，回抽，如无回血则可缓慢注入维生素 B_{12} 注射液，每穴 0.1mg。左右穴交替操作。

疗程：每天 1 次，左右穴交替，10 次为 1 个疗程。

注意事项：穴位注射当天局部避水，避免热敷；注射局部吸收不良时，可待吸收完全后再行治疗。

『推荐』

顽固性失眠建议配合维生素 B_{12} 注射液穴位注射。[GRADE 2D]

8.5 同行专家审定会意见

同行专家审定会是针对推荐方案可行性的再审阶段，会上专家提出的意见主要包括：①对于推荐方案下的证据应当给出相应的解释，以方便使用者理解。②建议将"泻阳跷，补阴跷"法写进推荐方案。③注意事项的内容需要进行适当调整。

根据上述意见，最终修改确定以下推荐方案。

8.5.1 毫针刺法

毫针刺法以改善全身气血状态为主要作用，因此在改善失眠患者整体睡眠质量方面（包括睡眠质量、入睡时间、睡眠时间、睡眠效率、睡眠障碍、催眠药物应用、日间功能障碍）效果显著，尤其在改善患者日间觉醒状态方面疗效突出。研究表明，毫针刺法的疗效可优于某些西药[34-37]，也可达到与中草药相当[38]的效果。

取穴（均双侧取穴）：①主穴：神门、四神聪、三阴交。②配穴：风池、太阳、本神。

辨证：肝郁化火型配太冲、肝俞、行间；肝郁痰热型配太冲、足三里；阴虚火旺型配心俞、肾俞、太溪、郄门；心脾两虚型配心俞、脾俞；心虚胆怯型配心俞、胆俞、丘墟；气滞血瘀型配太冲、血海、气海、肝俞、心俞。

操作方法：四神聪平刺，针尖方向朝向百会；本神向后平刺。其余腧穴均采用常规针刺法。针刺得气后，主、配穴均使用平补平泻法，辨证取穴根据证型行相应补泻手法，行针1分钟后留针。

疗程：每次留针30分钟，每周5次，10次为1个疗程，疗程之间间隔3天。

注意事项：临床应用时可于主穴适当配合使用电针（疏波）。

『推荐』

在改善失眠患者整体睡眠质量，尤其是日间觉醒状态方面，推荐使用结合脏腑辨证的毫针刺法。[GRADE 1B]

针对本方案，共有相关支撑文献57篇，经综合分析，形成证据体发现，局部安神穴与脏腑辨证结合可以有效提高患者整体睡眠质量，且在改善其日间觉醒状态方面疗效突出。本方案支撑证据数量较大，偏倚风险较低，经GRADE评价、专家共识后，因其文献设计质量、一致性及精确性高，最终证据体质量等级为中。

8.5.2 耳穴压丸法

耳穴压丸疗法能够平衡大脑皮层的兴奋与抑制，从而使皮层的功能活动趋于正常。因此，其疗效主要体现在改善患者睡眠时间、睡眠质量方面，其对于睡眠其他方面的改善尚少有研究。另外，在失眠治疗中，常规针刺结束后采用耳穴压丸的方式，在补充针灸治疗的基础上，更能给予皮层持久的小剂量刺激，更符合失眠的疾病特点。

取穴：①主穴：神门、皮质下、交感、内分泌、枕。②配穴：心、肾。

辨证：肝郁化火型配肝、胆；阴虚火旺型配肾、肝；心脾两虚型配脾、心、胃；心虚胆怯型配心、胆。

操作方法：针刺结束后，将王不留行籽（或磁珠）贴于0.5cm×0.5cm的医用胶布中央，耳穴常规消毒后，将粘有王不留行籽（或磁珠）的胶布贴在以上耳穴，并适度按压，使耳穴有胀、热、微痛感，每晚睡前按1次，约5分钟，以耳郭微红、微热为度，隔天换贴1次，双耳交替。

疗程：常规针灸治疗后进行，每3天更换1次，4次为1个疗程。

注意事项：①耳穴压丸疗法一般作为毫针刺法的延续治疗方法，单独使用疗效有限；只有短期或者轻度失眠患者单独使用可获较满意疗效。②如果耳穴按压后疼痛较剧烈，睡前可将其除去，防止因疼痛而影响睡眠。

『推荐』

> 在改善失眠患者睡眠时间和睡眠质量方面，建议使用耳穴压丸法。其中，慢性失眠建议将其作为毫针刺法的补充疗法；急性或亚急性失眠建议单独使用。[GRADE 2C]

针对本方案，共有相关支撑文献 8 篇，经综合分析，形成证据体发现，通过对相应耳穴的刺激来平衡大脑皮层的兴奋与抑制作用，对于改善失眠患者的睡眠时间、睡眠质量有较好的临床疗效。本方案形成时间较短，缺乏古代证据支撑，且证据数量不多，偏倚风险相对较高，但此方案众多的现代医家经验支撑，因此经 GRADE 评价、专家共识后，因其文献设计质量、一致性、精确性不高，但专家经验支撑力强，最终证据体质量等级为低。

8.5.3 头穴透刺法

透刺法作为平刺或斜刺的延伸应用，是通经行气、增强刺激的一种重要手法。将其应用于头部腧穴，在增强腧穴本身镇静安神作用的同时，可以有效疏通头部郁阻的经脉，因此更适用于伴有日间功能障碍的失眠患者，在改善其睡眠时间和睡眠质量的同时，可以有效提高日间活动效率。相关研究表明其疗效可优于毫针刺法[39]。

取穴：①主穴：前神聪透神庭、左右头临泣透左右神聪、后神聪透强间。②配穴：络却透通天、承光透曲差。

操作方法：针刺方向，由前神聪进针，平刺透向神庭；由头临泣进针，平刺透向同侧神聪；由后神聪进针，平刺透向强间。采用直径 0.35～0.40mm、长度 40～50mm 的毫针，针身与头皮呈 15°角，快速刺入头皮下，当针尖到达帽状腱膜下层，指下感到阻力减小时，将针与头皮平行，继续捻转进针，各穴进针深度 1～1.5 寸，然后快速小幅度左右捻针，每针行针约 1 分钟，取得较强针感后留针。

疗程：每次留针 30 分钟，每天 1 次，5 次为 1 个疗程，疗程之间间隔 2 天。

注意事项：临床应用时，头穴透刺作为主要治疗方法，需同时根据患者病情，辨证加用其他腧穴，针刺方法采用常规刺法。

『推荐』

> 伴有日间功能障碍的失眠患者，建议使用以头部安神腧穴透刺法为主，兼顾脏腑辨证的针刺疗法。[GRADE 2C]

针对本方案，共有相关支撑文献 3 篇，经综合分析，形成证据体发现，通过对头部局部腧穴进行透刺，不仅能够加强镇静安神作用，而且能够增加其疏通头部经气的功效，对于伴有日间功能障碍的失眠患者更加适用。本方案虽然支撑证据少，但存在质量相对较高的证据[11]，同时在专家共识阶段也得到专家一致支持，因此经 GRADE 评价、专家共识后，因其文献设计质量较高，一致性、精确性不高，但专家经验支撑力较高，最终证据体质量等级为低。

8.5.4 跷脉补泻法

由于人体的睡眠与阴阳跷脉的平衡有密切关系，因此，泻阳跷、补阴跷，使得阴阳达到平衡，就成为一种重要的治疗方法。其中，泻阳跷（申脉）可以有效改善觉醒时间、觉醒次数和深睡眠状况；而补阴跷（照海）则可以有效改善入睡困难的情况，二者侧重点有异。跷脉补泻法为泻阳跷和补阴跷的结合运用，在实际应用中需要根据患者病情的不同，酌情使用。

取穴：申脉、照海。

操作方法：患者仰卧位，针具、腧穴常规消毒后，先针照海，行捻转补法；再针申脉，行捻转泻法。

疗程：每次留针 30 分钟，每天 1 次，10 次为 1 个疗程，疗程之间间隔 3 天。

注意事项：①此方法需在明辨阴阳侧重的基础上灵活使用，且通常可与常规针刺法合用。②此方法中的两穴在针刺时容易有放电感出现，从而增加患者的紧张心理，因此在治疗前需要做好相应的告知和解释工作。③此方法用穴少，身体虚弱及惧怕针刺者可考虑使用。

『推荐』

> 在改善入睡困难、觉醒问题及深睡眠缺少方面，建议使用跷脉补泻法。身体虚弱及惧怕针刺的失眠患者建议使用本方法。[GRADE 2D]

针对本方案，共有相关支撑文献 7 篇，经综合分析，形成证据体发现，本方案通过泻阳跷、补阴跷，能够达到平衡阴阳的作用，从而可以针对性地改善患者入睡困难、觉醒问题、深睡眠缺少等问题。本方案证据数量不多，且 GRADE 评价级别极低，虽然专家共识一致性较高，可以对方案进行推荐，但无法提高其证据级别，因此，本方案最终证据体质量等级为极低。

8.5.5 皮肤针法

运用皮肤针治疗失眠，主要通过刺激膀胱经第一侧线及督脉来达到调整脏腑功能、疏达任督脉气的作用，除了能有效改善睡眠质量外，还能有效缩短患者入睡时间。研究表明，本疗法单独使用时可达到与某些西药相当的疗效[36]。此疗法突出优势在于不易产生耐药性及不良反应。

取穴：背部足太阳膀胱经第一、二侧线及督脉。

操作方法：患者俯卧位，沿膀胱经第一、二侧线由上向下，督脉由下向上进行叩击，每次叩击之间距离为 0.5cm，反复叩击 5 分钟，以皮肤潮红为度。膀胱经第一、二侧线实证可叩至皮肤微出血。

疗程：每次治疗 15～20 分钟，隔天 1 次，10 次为 1 个疗程。

注意事项：①此疗法可单独使用，也可作为针刺的配合疗法。②如叩刺出血，嘱患者 24 小时针孔避水，防止感染。

『推荐』

> 在改善失眠患者入睡困难方面，建议使用膀胱经及督脉皮肤针疗法；也可作为毫针刺法的配合疗法。[GRADE 2D]

针对本方案，共有相关支撑文献 7 篇，经综合分析，形成证据体发现，通过对膀胱、督脉的皮部进行刺激，不仅能够调整相应脏腑的功能，更能有效调顺督脉经气，从而改善患者睡眠质量，尤其是解决入睡困难的问题。本方案证据数量不多，偏倚风险较高，GRADE 评价级别为极低，虽然有专家经验证据支持，且专家共识一致性较高，可以对方案进行推荐，但无法提高其证据级别，因此，本方案最终证据体质量等级为极低。

8.5.6 穴位注射法

穴位注射将针刺、药理、药水对腧穴的渗透刺激作用结合在一起发挥综合效果，对于某些顽固性疾病效果可靠。主要用作顽固性失眠的辅助疗法。但目前尚无有力证据证明其与其他疗法在疗效方面的优劣关系。

取穴：风池、心俞。

药物：维生素 B_{12} 注射液。

操作方法：在上述腧穴注射，局部出现酸、麻、胀或放射感后，回抽，如无回血则可缓慢注入维生素 B_{12} 注射液，每穴 0.1mg。左右穴交替进行。

疗程：每天 1 次，左右穴交替进行，10 次为 1 个疗程。

注意事项：①穴位注射当天局部避水，避免热敷。②注射局部吸收不良时，可待吸收完全后再行治疗。

　　『推荐』

　　顽固性失眠建议配合维生素 B_{12} 注射液穴位注射。[GRADE 2D]

　　针对本方案，共有相关支撑文献10篇，经综合分析，形成证据体发现，穴位注射法通过综合腧穴、药物等作用，对于顽固性失眠可以产生较好的治疗效果，因此可以作为顽固性失眠的辅助治疗方法。本方案证据数量虽然较多，但偏倚风险较高，GRADE 评价级别为极低，虽然有一定数量的专家共识，但无法提高其证据级别，因此，本方案最终证据体质量等级为极低。

9　会议纪要

9.1　2013 年针灸临床实践指南项目审查会会议纪要

　　时间：2013 年9 月28 日。

　　地点：成都。

　　参会人员：国家中医药管理局、中国针灸学会的有关领导，以及全国针灸行业的科、教、研各方面共26 名专家出席了会议，此外，还有20 余名标准及指南起草单位的代表参加了会议。会议由中国针灸学会会长，全国针灸标准化技术委员会、中国针灸学会标准化工作委员会（以下简称"两针标委会"）主任委员刘保延主持，刘炜宏副主任委员、余曙光副主任委员分别担任28 日上午和下午两个时间段的审查专家组组长。

　　会议内容：

　　国家中医药管理局政策法规与监督司查德忠司长到会并做了重要讲话。查司长在讲话中指出，标准化工作是国家中医药管理局法监司的工作重点，受到各方面的重视，局里已陆续出台一系列关于标准化工作的意义、规划及管理办法的文件以指导相关工作，同时已得到中央财政设中医标准化专款支持标准化项目。查司长鼓励针灸行业继续积极开展标准化工作，争取长久进展，他特别强调，要重视针灸标准体系和针灸标准化支撑体系的构建，要将针灸标准的制定与应用相结合，将标准的评价与应用相结合，要积极推进针灸标准化培训工作。在讲话最后，查司长提出了四点建议：一是要继续完善针灸标准化体系框架；二是要加强标准通则的制定；三是要围绕针灸临床实践来制定标准；四是要夯实针灸标准制定的基础。

　　中国针灸学会会长刘保延代表学会及两针标委会介绍了参加本次审查会的2 项针灸国家标准、1 项针灸学会标准以及15 项针灸临床实践指南项目的实施情况。在两针标委会的组织下，该18 项标准（指南）的编制过程，严格遵循国家标准化管理委员会及中国针灸学会有关规定。目前，各项目组已对标准（指南）草案在全国范围内广泛征求意见，在今年6 月份召开的两针标委会2013 年年会上，该18 项标准（指南）草案已通过初审。本次会议受国家中医药管理局委托，由两针标委会组织专家对标准（指南）送审稿进行审查。刘保延会长特别强调，临床实践指南是未来针灸标准化工作的重点，其性质更加贴近临床，其研制目的是为临床疗效和质量提供保障，所以，本次审订会上，针灸临床实践指南的评审重点是推荐方案的实用性。刘保延会长特请本次审查委员会专家严格把关，以确保标准（指南）的质量，他希望没有通过审查的项目起草单位能够做好修改和完善工作。

　　本次审查会对提交大会的2 项针灸国家标准、1 项学会标准及15 项针灸临床实践指南进行了审议，根据专家评审意见及专家投票情况得出评审结果：通过国家标准1 项、学会标准1 项、行业指南6 项；建议修改后函审的行业指南3 项；建议修改后会审的国家标准1 项；未通过的行业指南6 项。具体情况如下：

　　（1）审议通过的项目

　　专家审查委员会审查通过了由全国针灸标准化技术委员会起草的针灸国家标准《针灸临床治疗指南制定及评估规范》，由湖北中医药大学起草的中国针灸学会标准《针刀基本技术操作规范》，由中国中医科学院广安门医院起草的《慢性便秘针灸临床实践指南》和《腰痛针灸临床实践指南》，由北京中医药大学东直门医院起草的《原发性痛经针灸临床实践指南》，由成都中医药大学起草的《坐骨神经痛针灸临床实践指南》，由中国中医科学院针灸研究所起草的《失眠针灸临床实践指南》和《支气管哮喘（成人）针灸临床实践指南》。

（2）修改后函审的项目

由中国中医科学院针灸研究所起草的《肩周炎针灸临床实践指南》、由天津中医药大学起草的《膝骨性关节炎针灸临床实践指南》以及由北京中医药大学东直门医院起草的《过敏性鼻炎针灸临床实践指南》3项指南，建议按照评审意见修订后再行函审。

（3）修改后会审的项目

由南京中医药大学起草的针灸国家标准《针灸门诊服务规范》，建议按照评审意见修订后再行会审。

（4）未通过的项目

由安徽中医学院附属针灸医院起草的《神经根型颈椎病针灸临床实践指南》、由天津中医药大学起草的《慢性萎缩性胃炎针灸临床实践指南》、由南京中医药大学起草的《突发性耳聋针灸临床实践指南》和《单纯性肥胖病针灸临床实践指南》、由浙江中医药大学附属医院起草的《原发性三叉神经痛针灸临床实践指南》以及由陕西中医学院起草的《糖尿病周围神经病变针灸临床实践指南》6项指南课题未通过审查。未通过审查的课题组按照评审意见继续修改和完善指南草案，由两针标委会秘书处另行安排验收审查。

最后，专家审查委员会提出，对于审议通过的标准，还需要对其内容及形式进行一致性修改，各标准起草单位应按照本次会议审查意见进行修改后，形成标准报批稿，上报两针标委会秘书处，经收集、整理、审核后，上报有关部门批准、发布。

《失眠针灸临床实践指南》（送审稿）专家审查意见

2013年9月28日，全国针灸标准化技术委员会、中国针灸学会标准化工作委员会在成都组织召开了"2013年针灸标准及临床实践指南项目审查会"，会上审查了《失眠针灸临床实践指南》（送审稿）。以余曙光为组长的22人专家组经过认真评议形成如下意见：本标准针对失眠针灸临床实践，通过收集整理失眠针灸临床实践和科研的相关文献资料、调研分析、专家论证，以古今文献、临床实践为依据，详细规定了该指南简介、疾病概述、临床特点、诊断标准、治疗概况、针灸治疗、推荐方案、附件等方面，形成了失眠针灸临床实践指南，并广泛征求专家意见，合理处理和分析相关意见，达成了共识。

专家组一致认为本针灸临床实践指南编写方法符合标准化的有关规定，资料完整，用语确切，格式规范；指南框架及内容系统实用，具有科学性和可行性；失眠针灸临床治疗推荐方案合理，具备公认性和适用性；规定的针灸临床实践指南要求符合当前的科技水平和发展方向。

专家提出如下修订建议：

（1）关于推荐方案

①推荐意见中并未阐明推荐理由，未阐明推荐方案能解决什么临床具体问题。

②去掉新药使用的指导方案，强调治疗方法的针对性，不建议依据中药新药临床指导原则。

③应介绍每个治疗方案在什么情况下应用。

④健康教育是针灸医生不可忽视的、与临床疗效密切相关的因素。

（2）关于针灸治疗

①P12取穴原则、治疗原则（6.6.1.2）方面的语言调整。

②"安眠穴"推荐为主穴；照海、申脉的应用；顽固性失眠不建议穴位注射；头穴透刺法要明确

其疗效特点，如起效快。

③穴位埋线疗法是治疗失眠的有效方法，建议纳入。

④出现频次高的腧穴间相配是否就是最优？

⑤毫针6.6.1.1，其疗效优于西药，下结论应慎重；6.1中"特点"内容未及，宜补；"原则"稍笼统。

⑥建议使用针灸临床实际辨证取穴，避免套用中医临床诊断分型。

⑦缺少特征性分析，需要指出治疗特点。

（3）关于诊断标准

①观察诊断的客观评价，可使用一些量表，建议主客观观察结合。

②4.2中医诊断标准及分型：1994年制定的标准，是否有更新？

（4）其他

①语言应规范、严谨，应使用标准用词，如"应、可、宜"。如推荐方案，宜用"可推荐"，而不宜用"建议推荐"。

②应注意文本各章节、段之间详略得当。

③各种方法的概述应删除，不应给予定义式描述。

审查组同意该指南通过审查。建议根据专家意见修改后，以行业标准上报审批。

全国针灸标准化技术委员会

中国针灸学会标准化工作委员会

2013年9月28日

附：《失眠针灸临床实践指南》项目评审专家名单

序号	姓名	职称/职务	工作单位
1	刘保延	副院长	中国中医科学院
2	刘炜宏	编审	中国中医科学院针灸所
3	文碧玲	教授	中国针灸学会
4	武晓冬	副研究员	中国中医科学院针灸所
5	余曙光	副校长/研究员	成都中医药大学
6	郭 义	教授	天津中医药大学
7	杨 骏	院长/教授	安徽中医学院
8	杨华元	教授	上海中医药大学
9	房繁恭	研究员	中国中医科学院针灸所
10	储浩然	主任医师	安徽省针灸医院
11	赵 宏	主任医师	中国中医科学院广安门医院
12	石 现	主任医师	解放军总医院针灸科
13	王富春	院长/教授	长春中医药大学针灸推拿学院
14	王麟鹏	主任医师	首都医科大学附属北京中医医院
15	贾春生	主任医师/教授	河北医科大学中医学院
16	余晓阳	主任医师	重庆市中医院

序号	姓名	职称/职务	工作单位
17	高希言	教授	河南中医学院
18	常小荣	教授	湖南中医药大学
19	吕明庄	主任医师	贵州省贵阳医学院附属医院
20	王玲玲	院长/教授	南京中医药大学
21	宣丽华	主任医师	浙江中医药大学附属第一医院
22	翟 伟	教授	内蒙古医科大学中医学院

9.2 本《指南》推荐方案专家论证会会议纪要

2014 年 3 月 20 日，由刘保延、武晓冬、刘志顺、王麟鹏、赵宏等针灸临床专家及 6 个针灸临床实践指南主研人员参加的第二批针灸临床实践指南推荐方案专家论证会在中国中医科学院召开，经过专家论证，对本指南进行认真论证，形成意见如下：

（1）指南中所用术语应与其他各课题组间统一。

（2）具体推荐方案中的"注意事项"应当写该方案治疗该疾病时针对性的注意事项，整个针灸疗法的共性的注意事项不应赘述。

（3）对指南推荐方案中的证据可以进行进一步详细解释。

（4）针灸治疗特点部分应当进一步充实，主要内容应当是对针灸治疗失眠意义重大，但是在推荐方案中不便出现的内容。

（5）建议将申脉、照海的应用纳入推荐中，虽然其支撑证据级别较低，但临床应用较广泛，专家共识级别较高，因此，可以予以推荐。

最终，各课题组的推荐方案和意见均已通过专家的讨论和修正。总课题组建议下一步工作安排：各临床指南课题组针对专家给出的意见就推荐方案进行进一步的修改和完善；针对各课题组提出的统一针灸临床专业术语和指南定稿格式的问题，总课题组经商议和明确后尽快给予回复；时间紧迫，要求各课题组在两周之内完成指南的最终定稿。

———————